Pocket Examiner in Surgery

Pocket Examiner
in
Surgery

John Northover MS FRCS
Consultant Surgeon
St Mark's Hospital, London
Senior Lecturer, Department of Surgery
The Medical College, St Bartholomew's Hospital

Tom Treasure MD MS FRCS
Consultant Cardiothoracic Surgeon,
The Middlesex Hospital

With contributions from:

Matthew Fletcher
Senior Surgical Registrar,
King's College Hospital

John Dixon
Consultant Orthopaedic Surgeon
Winford Orthopaedic Hospital, Bristol

Michael Bridger
Consultant ENT Surgeon
Plymouth General Hospital

Paul Hunter
Consultant Ophthalmic Surgeon,
King's College Hospital

Kenneth Lindsay
Consultant Neurosurgeon,
Royal Free Hospital

Churchill Livingstone 🚢
Edinburgh London Melbourne and New York 1986

CHURCHILL LIVINGSTONE
Medical Division of Longman Group UK Limited

Distributed in the United States of America by
Churchill Livingstone Inc., 650 Avenue of the Americas,
New York, N.Y. 10011, and by associated companies,
branches and representatives throughout the world.

© John Northover and Tom Treasure 1984

All rights reserved. No part of this publication
may be reproduced, stored in a retrieval system,
or transmitted in any form or by any means,
electronic, mechanical, photocopying, recording or
otherwise, without the prior permission of the
publishers (Churchill Livingstone, Robert Stevenson
House, 1–3 Baxter's Place, Leith Walk,
Edinburgh EH1 3AF), or a license permitting
restricted copying in the United Kingdom issued
by the Copyright Licensing Agency Ltd,
90 Tottenham Court Road, London, W1P 9HE.

First published 1984 (Pitman Publishing Ltd)
  Reprinted 1984
  Reprinted 1986 (Churchill Livingstone)
  Reprinted 1988
  Reprinted 1989
  Reprinted 1993

ISBN 0-443-03654-3

British Library Cataloguing in Publication Data
A catalogue record for this book is available from the
British Library.

Library of Congress Cataloging in Publication Data
Northover, John
    Pocket examiner in surgery.
    1. Surgery Examinations, questions, etc.
    I. Treasure, Tom.   II. Fletcher, Matthew.   III. Title.
    [DNLM: 1. Surgery—examination questions.   WO 18
N876p] RD37.2.N67 1984   617'.0076   84–9530

Produced by Longman Singapore Publishers Pte Ltd
Printed in Singapore

Contents

Foreword

by Professor Harold Ellis, DM MCh FRCS
Surgical Unit, Westminster Hospital, London

I was greatly honoured when I was approached by John Northover and Tom Treasure to prepare a foreword for this interesting book, and still more delighted after I had had the opportunity of reading it through in manuscript.

I think I can describe myself, without any fear of contradiction, as an experienced examiner. Over the past quarter of a century, I have examined medical students in seven Universities in this country and another half a dozen overseas, stretching from Hong Kong to the West Indies via Ethiopia. I believe I know every trick of the trade among my examiner colleagues and I am acquainted with every device invented by the students to ensure that they defeat us! Examinations are used as an educative force. Examiners know that students will learn what they expect will crop up in the examinations, and, very wisely, that they will leave out those topics they expect, or hope, the examiners to omit. It therefore behoves the examiners to ensure that their questions are relevant to the sort of knowledge their students should acquire during their clinical years.

Going through the questions in this pocket examiner, I was delighted to see many of my old friends and also to find some that were refreshingly new. I was interested to find the wide range of subjects covered in a surprisingly short space. Checking the questions against the specimen answers, I was quite prepared to give the authors, and their five collaborators, very high marks indeed!

It would seem to me that the revision student could either use this book alone, reading the question, giving a reply, then checking this against the text, or better, working in a group and taking it in turn to answer the question and to consult the crib. But whichever technique is used, I commend this volume to my friends the surgical finalists and wish them good luck in their encounters with the examiners.

Harold Ellis

Preface

Oral examination is a traditional and vital part of the
assessment of medical students throughout their education;
it allows the examiners not only to test knowledge but also
to form an opinion about the candidate's ability to marshal
his thoughts logically and rapidly in trying conditions. It is
this immediacy that makes the clinical and viva voce parts
of the final examination particularly worrying to students.
There is only limited time available with teachers to
practise one-to-one examination technique, so generations of
students have sat at home, text books on their knees,
quizzing each other. Conventional texts do not lend
themselves to this process, so the authors have striven to fill
the gap. We have presented surgery in an oral question and
answer form, precisely as used by examiners, to help
students improve their fluency and test their knowledge in a
structured way.

There are some important rules to be remembered in oral
examinations:

1 Listen carefully to the question—it's the only one the
   examiner wants answered!
2 Silence scores no points—you must start answering
   quickly, while remembering that you should first decide
   on the nub of the answer, and aim to get it across in your
   opening sentence.
3 Do not get bogged down in rarities and areas of
   controversy unless you are very sure of yourself—the
   examiner will know more about them than you do!

These skills only come with practice: we hope that this
volume will make it easier for students to acquire them
while also picking up a few extra facts. The questions and
answers have been prepared by a group of young surgeons
who are regularly involved in teaching and yet can still
remember what it is like to be on the receiving end.

JMAN
TT

Acknowledgements

We would like to thank Katharine Watts and Peter Abrahams for approaching us to write this book. Sue Stannard's word processing skills made the task of editing bearable. Our wives and sons tolerated many weekends of writing and we appreciate their forbearance.

1   Questions

'On the spot'

1   Imagine that you are faced with a 35 year old Scottish lorry driver who has been struck down suddenly with epigastric pain which rapidly became generalized. On examination he is cold, sweaty and has abdominal rigidity and no bowel sounds.
    What would be your immediate management?

2   A child has had a tonsillectomy earlier in the day and you are called by the nurses because they suspect postoperative bleeding.
    What do you look for?

3   Imagine you are a medical houseman. A patient of yours, admitted four days ago with a myocardial infarct, develops generalized abdominal pain with guarding and loss of bowel sounds.
    What do you suspect?

4   A 75 year old lady complains of a complete and sudden loss of her right vision two days previously associated with right-sided headaches for some weeks. She also admits to weight loss, anorexia and tenderness of her scalp while combing her hair.
    What steps would you take to try to ensure that she keeps her left vision?

5   You are a surgical houseman. The casualty officer refers a two year old who has swallowed a penny. X-rays confirm that it is below the diaphragm.
    What are you going to do about it?

6   An obese, middle-aged man with a history of atheromatous disease presents with a 24 hour history of severe back pain. He is pale, clammy and shocked. He is too obese to confirm by palpation your suspicion of a leaking aortic aneurysm.
    What would be your further management?

7   Imagine that, as a casualty officer, you are faced with a 64 year old man who presents in a shocked state, having developed severe left posterior chest pain while vomiting at the end of a long evening's eating and drinking. You place a calming hand on his shoulder

and discover crepitus, most marked in the supraclavicular fossa.

What has happened to this man? What will the surgeons do for him?

8   A fat woman presents with obvious jaundice, right hypochondrial pain and fever with rigors.

What is the most likely diagnosis?

9   A 35 year old alcoholic has had a large haematemesis.

What are the likely causes and how would you make the precise diagnosis?

10   What should you do during the first 24 hours following the admission of a young man who has had three hours of excruciating right loin pain?

11   A patient who underwent an emergency gastrectomy for perforated gastric ulcer a week ago complains of lower chest pain on inspiration and pain in the left shoulder tip. On examination he is tender under the left costal margin and has a mild pyrexia.

What may be the diagnosis and what investigations should be performed?

12   A young woman of 20 gives a short history of profuse, bloody diarrhoea. On examination she has a slight temperature, there is tenderness in the left abdomen and fresh blood on rectal examination.

What is your differential diagnosis and what investigations would you arrange?

13   An old man with no past history except for rheumatoid arthritis presents with a history of vomiting a 'bucketful' of blood.

What are the principles of his management?

14   A patient with multiple injuries has a distending abdomen and frank blood is found on peritoneal lavage. However, he is unconscious due to a head injury.

Does this influence management of his abdomen?

15   A cyclist is brought into casualty after an apparently quite minor accident. By the time you see him he is breathless and panicking.

What is your immediate management?

16   A man of 60 is taken to his family doctor having, over a period of three days, suffered several episodes of slurred speech and confusion from each of which he has recovered.

What is the likely cause and what must the doctor do?

17 A four month old baby is brought in with a 24 hour history of intermittent screaming, pulling up of his knees, and the passage of blood and mucus per rectum.
   What is the most likely diagnosis and how would you confirm it?

18 Imagine that you have admitted a patient with acute pancreatitis who fails to improve as quickly as you might normally expect. Ten days after admission, with the amylase still at 2000, you feel a mass in the epigastrium.
   What do you think may be the problem? How will you confirm the diagnosis?

19 A quarryman, hurt in a rock fall, is brought to casualty. He has tried and failed to pass urine and has some blood at the urethral meatus.
   What do you do next?

20 How would you manage a 60 year old man who presents as an emergency with an episode of brisk, fresh bleeding per rectum?

21 A lady of 57 has become increasingly breathless and has had attacks of palpitations over the past few years. She now presents with a sudden onset of pain and weakness in both legs.
   What do you suspect has happened and how would you confirm it?

22 A previously fit 60 year old presents with weight loss, anorexia and recent, worsening dysphagia for solids.
   What may be wrong? How would you investigate this patient?

23 A 40 year old woman comes to you with a painful breast lump, apparently worried that she has breast cancer.
   What are you going to do for her?

24 An elderly patient with claudication gives a few hours' history of left abdominal pain and bloody diarrhoea.
   What do you think might be wrong with him?

25 A woman of 55 with griping central abdominal pain, diarrhoea, intermittent facial flushing and shortness of breath is exhibiting the typical features of a particular syndrome.
   What is it and what is the pathological basis of the features described?

26 A patient is admitted to casualty in coma following a road traffic accident.
   What are the priorities of assessment?

27 A young man, who fell on an iron spike injuring a buttock the day before, presents feeling ill and has crepitus around the wound.
What is the likely diagnosis and management?

28 A patient complains of a painful swelling below the angle of the jaw just before meals.
What is the likely cause?

The acute abdomen

General clinical features

29 What characteristics of an abdominal pain would suggest the presence of peritoneal inflammation?

30 What do we mean by 'peritonism'?

31 Can peritoneal inflammation ever produce pain at a non-abdominal site?

32 What are the four classical symptoms of intestinal obstruction?

33 What is the difference between faecal and faeculent vomiting?

34 What is the difference between tenderness and guarding in the abdomen?

35 Before palpating an acute abdomen, what abdominal signs should you *look* for?

36 Do you know of any non-abdominal conditions which can mimic 'the acute abdomen'?

37 What acute abdominal conditions can produce back pain?

38 What is rebound tenderness and how do you test for it?

Appendicitis

39 Do you know why acute appendicitis develops?

40 What are the typical symptoms and signs of appendicitis?

41 Why does the pain usually start centrally and later move to the right iliac fossa?

42 Where is McBurney's point? What is its significance?

43 Have you any idea what would happen if a patient with acute appendicitis were left untreated?

44 If a patient with a typical story of appendicitis is found to have a tender mass in the right iliac fossa, what may be going on?

45 If a patient develops a pyrexia following appendicectomy, what might the cause be?

46 If at operation for suspected appendicitis the appendix is found to be normal, what does the surgeon check for before closing the abdomen?

Biliary disease

47 What are the typical symptoms and signs of acute cholecystitis?

48 Have you ever seen a patient with biliary colic?
   What do you remember about the clinical presentation?

49 Do you know of any investigations to help us check the diagnosis of acute cholecystitis during the acute phase?
   When is such investigation particularly important?

50 When we diagnose acute cholecystitis we give intravenous fluids and nothing by mouth.
   Why?

51 What are the indications for urgent surgery in someone with acute cholecystitis?

52 Is ascending cholangitis a serious condition?
   How do we manage it?

53 What is gall-stone ileus?

Perforated peptic ulcer

54 What does a perforated duodenal ulcer look like at operation?
   Which part of the duodenum is usually involved?

55 Do you know whether the clinical picture presented by elderly patients with perforated ulcer differs from that seen in younger patients?

56 Which x-ray is the most useful in the diagnosis of perforation?

57 Are any investigations required before laparotomy in a patient who clinically appears to have perforated peptic ulcer but in whom no free gas is seen on x-ray?

58 What are the usual operations for perforated duodenal or gastric ulcer?

59 Have you any idea how to manage a perforated peptic ulcer in someone medically unfit for surgery?

60 Do you know of any drugs that predispose to perforated peptic ulcer?

Complications of diverticular disease

61 What is the difference between diverticulosis and diverticulitis?

62 What do we mean by 'left-sided appendicitis'?

63 How is acute diverticulitis diagnosed and managed?

64 What are the clinical features of pericolic abscess? How is it managed?

65 What sorts of peritonitis can result from the complications of diverticular disease?

66 What are the stages in the management of a patient with peritonitis due to perforated diverticular disease?

67 What is the prognosis in patients suffering from perforated diverticular disease?

Acute pancreatitis

68 What are the causes of acute pancreatitis?

69 What are the typical clinical features of this condition?

70 How do you confirm the diagnosis?

71 How would you manage a patient with this condition?

72 What is the prognosis in acute pancreatitis?

Vascular conditions

73 What part of the bowel is usually affected by embolic mesenteric infarction? Is this condition treatable?

74 Do you know how we tell whether ischaemic bowel is dead?

75 Why does ischaemic colitis usually affect the colon around the splenic flexure?

76 Does ischaemic colitis usually require operation?

Gynaecological emergencies

77 What gynaecological emergencies can mimic appendicitis?

78 Do you know how a ruptured ectopic pregnancy presents?

79 How would you distinguish between appendicitis and acute salpingitis?

Intestinal obstruction

80 What are the commonest causes of small bowel obstruction in adults?

81 Why do patients with distal small bowel obstruction become dehydrated, even before they have started vomiting?

82 What do we mean by reversed peristalsis?

83 What is closed loop obstruction?

84 What is subacute obstruction?

85 How do we go about deciding how much and what type of intravenous fluid replacement to give to a patient with intestinal obstruction?

86 What are the constituents of 'normal' saline?

87 What is Hartmann's solution?

88 How do we differentiate small bowel from large bowel in the abdominal x-rays of someone with intestinal obstruction?

89 Why do we bother to make this differentiation?

90 What blood tests would you order in someone with intestinal obstruction?

91 If you saw gas in the biliary tree on the x-rays of an old lady with unexplained small bowel obstruction, what might you suspect?

92 What sort of acid-base abnormality develops in intestinal obstruction?

93 What x-ray signs would indicate the presence of dead bowel in someone with intestinal obstruction?

94 What radiological investigations might you order in a child with suspected ileocolic intussusception?

95 What are the commonest abdominal operations leading to adhesions, and hence adhesive small bowel obstruction?

96 How do we decide if and when to operate on someone with small bowel obstruction due to adhesions?

97 Is visible peristalsis always pathological?

98 Are there any types of small bowel obstruction peculiar to patients who have previously undergone a gastrectomy?

99 Is there anything we can do to try to prevent further problems in someone who has had repeated bouts of small bowel obstruction?

100 What symptoms and signs suggest that someone with small bowel obstruction has developed strangulation of a bowel segment?

101 How do the symptoms of small and large bowel obstruction differ?

102 What is the commonest cause of large bowel obstruction?

103 What is spurious diarrhoea?

104 Are there any dangers in 'sitting on' a case of large bowel obstruction?

105 What is sigmoid volvulus?

106 How do we treat someone with intestinal obstruction due to sigmoid carcinoma?

107 What is pseudo-obstruction?

108 What is a 'string' carcinoma?

Abdominal trauma

109 What is the significance of finding tyre tread marks on the abdomen of a patient from a road traffic accident?

110 What is the likely cause of melaena in a patient who has become jaundiced several days following an untreated stab wound just above the right costal margin?

111 What symptoms and signs suggest the diagnosis of ruptured spleen?

112 Why does a chest wall injury in a road traffic accident patient make evaluation of abdominal signs more difficult?

113 Up to what level on the chest wall should penetrating injuries be regarded as having possibly entered the abdominal cavity?

114 What intra-abdominal organs are specially liable to injury in a patient wearing a seat-belt during a head-on collision?

115 What are the relative dangers of intra-abdominal visceral damage due to injuries produced by a knife, hand-gun and high-velocity rifle?

116 Following a stabbing, the victim is found at laparotomy to have a knife wound in the anterior wall of the stomach. The surgeon simply repairs this and closes the abdomen.
 He is likely to be re-operating soon — why?

117 What is a subcapsular haematoma of the spleen? What is its significance?

118 How can a crush injury to the abdomen result in severe mechanical respiratory embarrassment?

119 What is the most efficient investigation to confirm or exclude intraperitoneal haemorrhage?
 How exactly is this performed?

120 What are the radiological signs of a ruptured spleen?

121 What is the usefulness of inserting a probe into an abdominal stab wound to assess the depth of penetration?

122 What x-ray signs suggest a diaphragmatic rupture?

123 In which types of abdominal trauma is laparotomy mandatory?

124 How would you manage a patient admitted with abdominal trauma in whom laparotomy is not immediately indicated?

125 How do we manage penetrating wounds of the large bowel at laparotomy?

126 What antibiotics would you prescribe as part of the treatment of a patient with a stab wound involving the large bowel?

127 A patient who has received a stab wound to the abdomen is found at laparotomy to have a laceration of the right lobe of the liver.
 What surgical manoeuvres are likely to be considered?

General surgical care

Water, electrolytes and nutrition

128 What are the body's normal daily gains and losses of water?

129 How would you assess the water requirements of a patient in the first 24 hours after a routine abdominal operation?

130 You may have to repeat the exercise on a more complicated, critically ill patient.
   What other factors should be taken into account?

131 What is the normal 24 hour turnover of sodium?

132 How would you interpret a serum sodium of 124 mmol/litre?

133 What is the significance of a high serum sodium?

134 How much potassium is contained in the urine?

135 How might a low serum potassium occur?
   What are the possible consequences?

136 A patient's potassium rises to 6.8 mmol/litre after surgery.
   What are you going to do about it?

137 In a patient with intestinal obstruction and a Ryle's tube down, what approximate electrolyte composition would you expect in the aspirate?
   How would you take account of this in your fluid replacement?

138 How would you judge the appropriate intravenous replacement for the loss from a gastro-intestinal fistula?

139 What hazards may be encountered in the treatment of hypokalaemia?

140 In what chemical forms is calcium found in serum?

141 Suggest some causes for and consequences of hypercalcaemia.

142 Under what circumstances may magnesium deficiency occur?

143 What surgical problems may be encountered in a patient who has had difficulty taking an adequate diet in the pre-operative period?

144 If it proves necessary to maintain a patient by the intravenous route alone, what basic constituents should this diet contain?

145 What risks are entailed in this therapy?

Management of the circulation

146 What do you understand by the term 'shock'?

147 Define 'hypovolaemia' and explain how you would reach this diagnosis.

148 What solutions are available for expanding the circulation and what are their relative merits?

149 What information can you gain by measuring the central venous pressure?

150 How would you set about measuring the central venous pressure?

151 How would you define oliguria?

152 What immediate steps would you take to remedy oliguria?

153 What factors cause or contribute to the development of acute renal failure?

154 How would you manage this condition?

155 Soon after a major operation your patient is noted to have a diastolic blood pressure of 110 mmHg.
   How do you assess and manage this?

156 Summarize the potential hazards of blood transfusion.

157 The patient is bleeding excessively during surgery and you suspect a coagulopathy.
   How do you confirm and manage the problem?

Postoperative complications

158 List some possible causes of a pyrexia noted between three and ten days after surgery.

159 How would you investigate a low grade pyrexia during the week after surgery for which the cause is not obvious?

160 What are the implications of a swinging pyrexia during the second week after an abdominal operation?

161 What factors contribute to the occurrence of wound infections?

162 What organisms would you specifically enquire about in infection complicating a large bowel resection?

163 If you have located an abscess and know the organism, how would you treat it?

164 What pulmonary complications might be anticipated after major surgery?

165 What precautions can be taken to reduce the potential chest problems in a bronchitic undergoing abdominal surgery?

166 What is intrapulmonary shunting?
How would you recognize and deal with it?

167 In the second postoperative week a patient coughs up
some blood.
What steps would you take?

168 What is Virchow's triad?
How does it apply to the postoperative patient?

169 Why would you suspect and how would you confirm the
diagnosis of a deep vein thrombosis?

170 What are the typical clinical features of pulmonary
embolism?

171 How would you confirm the diagnosis?

172 What treatment is available?

173 How do we try to prevent thrombo-embolism?

174 If a myocardial infarction occurs under anaesthetic,
the typical clinical features are not seen.
How would you know it had happened?

175 The night of the operation a tachycardia is noted.
How would you decide what to do about it?

176 You are the only doctor at a cardiac arrest.
What are you going to do?

177 How would you deal with sudden profuse bleeding from
an abdominal drain?

'Lumps and bumps'

178 In your examination of a lump what physical features
would you note?

179 How would you elicit fluctuance?

180 What would you infer if the lump were tethered?

181 How would tensing the muscles in the region of a lump
help decide its anatomical position?

182 What features of a lump permit transillumination?

183 What general features would suggest bacterial
infection as the cause of a lump?

184 How is an abscess diagnosed and managed?

185 What is cellulitis and what organism is likely to be
responsible?

186 What is the difference between a boil and a carbuncle?

187 What is the likely nature of a soft, lobulated, subcutaneous lump?

188 What is Dercum's disease?

189 What are the typical clinical features of a sebaceous cyst?

190 What causes warts to come and go?

191 What is keloid?

192 Outline the essentials of the TNM classification of malignant tumours.

193 What changes in a mole make malignancy a possibility?

194 How would you confirm the diagnosis in a clinically suspected malignant melanoma?

195 What factors may predispose to squamous cell carcinoma?

196 Describe the clinical features of a rodent ulcer.

197 Give the differential diagnosis in a patient who is found to have enlarged axillary lymph nodes.

198 A patient reports that he develops a swelling in his neck immediately after eating.
   What might it be?

199 A group of enlarged nodes is found on one side of the neck.
   What are the possible diagnoses?

200 A recently noticed tender lump in the groin might be due to what?

201 What do you think was particularly important about the original description of Burkitt's tumour?

202 What are the causes of a tender scrotal swelling?

Hernia

203 What are the surface landmarks of the superficial inguinal ring?

204 What are the boundaries of the deep inguinal ring?

205 What structures constitute the spermatic cord?

206 What are the boundaries of the femoral canal?

207 Define the term 'hernia'.

208 What is the importance of the neck of a hernial sac?

209 What types of hernia occur in the groin?

210 Explain the exact meaning of the words 'direct' and 'indirect' in this context.

211 Can you give the relative frequency of the various types of groin hernia?

212 What would you include in the differential diagnosis of inguinoscrotal swellings in children?

213 Which inguinal herniae can be considered more likely to be congenital and which to be acquired?

214 How often are groin herniae bilateral?

215 On the grounds of probability alone, what type of groin hernia are you most likely to find in a woman?

216 Besides the groin, where else may an external hernia occur?

217 What is meant by the word 'exomphalos'?

218 What is the usual outcome of an umbilical hernia noted soon after birth?

219 What is the aetiology of incisional hernia and how may it be avoided?

220 What exactly is meant by the term 'herniotomy'?

221 What are the principles involved in the operation of herniorrhaphy?

222 Explain what is meant by a sliding hernia. What is its other name?

223 When might it be necessary to perform an orchidectomy to obtain satisfactory repair?

224 Is surgery always successful in the repair of inguinal hernia?

225 What methods can be used to repair an incisional hernia?

226 Define 'strangulation'.

227 Of the groin herniae, which are the more liable to strangulate?

228 What complications may occur with a femoral hernia?

229 Describe some eponymous herniae.

230 In what circumstances can strangulation occur without obstruction?

231 Under what circumstances would you consider it reasonable to manage a hernia with a truss?

232 What would be the result of an untreated, strangulated hernia?

Alimentary tract

The mouth and salivary glands

233 An old lady who has recently undergone major surgery complains of a sore mouth. On examination she has many white patches on the lining of the buccal cavity.
What is the diagnosis and management?

234 What are the typical symptoms and signs of cancer of the tongue?

234 Do you know any predisposing factors to cancer of the oral cavity?

236 What is a ranula?

237 An old man develops a painful, brawny red swelling on one side of his face in front of the ear several days after a major abdominal operation. What is the most likely diagnosis?
Why does this condition develop?

238 What nerves are liable to damage during surgery on the salivary glands?

239 Where do the parotid and submandibular salivary ducts open into the mouth?

240 Why is mumps parotitis so painful?

241 What are the various names of the commonest tumour of the parotid gland?
How is it treated?

242 What are the chances of recurrence after removal of a pleomorphic adenoma of the parotid?

243 Do stones ever form in the parotid duct?

244 What is thought to be the cause of salivary duct stones?

245 How do we manage a patient with a submandibular duct stone?

The oesophagus

246 What anatomical factors normally prevent reflux at the lower end of the oesophagus?

247 What is the structure of the oesophageal wall?

248 Define dysphagia. List some causes.

249 What is the difference between vomiting and regurgitation?

250 How can potassium therapy cause an oesophageal stricture?

251 Briefly, what do you know of the pathology of oesophageal cancer?

252 What sorts of treatment are available for carcinoma of the oesophagus?

253 What is the prognosis in patients with carcinoma of the oesophagus?

254 What is heartburn?

255 What sorts of hiatal hernia do you know?
   How may their presentations differ?

256 What complications can develop in patients with sliding hiatal hernia?

257 Can you list the forms of treatment available for hiatal hernia?
   What are their indications?

258 What do you know about achalasia?

259 Where exactly do benign oesophageal strictures usually occur?
   How are they managed?

260 What forms of treatment are available for bleeding oesophageal varices?

The stomach

261 What structures related to the stomach may become involved by direct spread of a gastric cancer?

262 What is the blood supply of the stomach?

263 What parts of the stomach produce gastrin, acid and pepsin?

264 What are the functions of the stomach?

265 What stimuli induce gastric acid secretion?

266 How can we reduce gastric acid secretion?

267 What are the different ways in which gastric cancer can present?

268 Do you know any factors which predispose to gastric cancer?

269 What is linitis plastica?

270 Briefly, what operations are available for gastric cancer?

271 Can we offer patients with gastric cancer a good chance of cure?

272 Why do patients with gastric ulcer tend to lose weight?

273 In a patient with a gastric ulcer what is the significance of back pain?

274 Why should gastroscopy be mandatory in the investigation of a gastric ulcer patient?

275 How should we manage a patient with an apparently benign, uncomplicated gastric ulcer?

276 What are the complications of gastric ulcer?

277 What radiological features suggest a gastric ulcer might be malignant?

278 What is erosive gastritis?
    What are its causes?

279 How do we manage a patient who is shown endoscopically to be bleeding from erosive gastritis?

280 What are the important causes of upper gastro-intestinal bleeding?

281 Why do most clinicians prefer to endoscope patients with upper gastro-intestinal bleeding soon after admission?
    Does this investigation affect mortality?

282 What operations are available for bleeding peptic ulcer (gastric or duodenal)?

283 What is the overall mortality today for acute upper gastro-intestinal bleeding?
    Which lesions are particularly dangerous?

The duodenum

284 What is the duodenal cap?

285 What structures may be involved when a duodenal ulcer penetrates through the wall?

286 What hormones does the duodenal mucosa secrete?
    What stimulates their production, and what are their actions?

287 How is the duodenal mucosa normally protected from acid/peptic digestion?

288 How does a duodenal ulcer usually present?

289 What is waterbrash?

290 How do we definitively diagnose an active duodenal ulcer?

291 Having proven the presence of a simple duodenal ulcer how do we normally manage the patient?

292 What do we mean by failed medical management in a patient with duodenal ulcer?

293 What are the indications for surgery in duodenal ulcer?

294 What operations are available for duodenal ulcer?

295 Why do we not normally perform a pyloroplasty with highly selective vagotomy?

296 What are the long-term complications of duodenal ulcer surgery?

The pancreas

297 What is the nerve supply of the pancreas?
When is this clinically important?

298 How is pancreatic exocrine function controlled?

299 How does the presentation of cancer of the head of the pancreas differ from that of cancer of the body or tail?

300 What extra-abdominal manifestations of pancreatic cancer do you know?

301 Can we prove a diagnosis of pancreatic cancer without laparotomy?

302 What treatment is available for cancer of the pancreas?

303 What is chronic pancreatitis?

304 What forms of treatment are available for chronic pancreatitis?

305 What is a pancreatic pseudocyst?
How is it managed?

The liver

306 Where is the dividing line between the right and the left lobes of the liver?
Is it clinically important?

307 What structures are in danger of accidental damage during an attempted liver biopsy?

308 How can we diagnose liver secondaries?

309 Are liver secondaries treatable?
    If so, how?

310 What are the conditions known to predispose to primary hepatocellular carcinoma?

311 What liver condition is particularly related to contact with sheep?

312 Which tropical bowel infection sometimes produces a special type of liver abscess?
    How is this abscess treated?

313 Who gets liver abscesses in this country?

314 How can we treat a unilocular liver abscess?

315 What are oesophageal varices?

The biliary tree

316 What anatomical structures are at risk of accidental damage during cholecystectomy?
    How do such injuries occur?

317 What is the anatomy of the lower end of the common bile duct?

318 What are the functions of bile?

319 What abnormalities of bile lead to stone formation?

320 Can you describe the typical 'gallstone patient' and her symptoms?

321 What do we call the other clinical presentations of gallstone disease?

322 What investigations help confirm the clinical suspicion of gall bladder disease?
    How are they performed?

323 Which patients are most and least helped by cholecystectomy for gallstones?

324 What are the major steps in routine cholecystectomy?

325 What is operative cholangiography?

326 Can stones be 'removed' from the gall bladder other than by surgery?

327 What do we mean by obstructive jaundice?
    What are the causes?

328 Why do patients with obstructive jaundice often complain of itching?
   How can it be treated?

329 How do we confirm obstructive jaundice biochemically?

330 What is a percutaneous transhepatic cholangiogram?
   When is it useful?

331 What is the hepatorenal syndrome and how do we try to prevent it?

332 What is a T-tube?
   How do we manage it postoperatively?

333 What can we do if a T-tube cholangiogram shows retained stones in the common bile duct?

334 What is a mucocele of the gall bladder?

335 What are the causes of bile duct strictures?

336 What do you know about gall bladder cancer?

The spleen

337 What organs may be damaged during splenectomy?

338 What physical signs suggest an abdominal mass is an enlarged spleen?

339 What are the commonest causes of splenomegaly in Britain?

340 What are the usual indications for splenectomy?

341 What are the early and late complications of splenectomy?

342 What are splenunculi and what is their importance?

The small bowel

343 What major artery supplies the small bowel?
   What is the course of the trunk of this vessel?

344 What are the physiological consequences of resection of the distal 2 ft of ileum?

345 How does Crohn's disease affecting the small bowel usually present?

346 What are the extra-abdominal manifestations of Crohn's disease?

347 What are the radiological characteristics of Crohn's disease?

348 What are the indications for surgery in Crohn's disease?

349 What are the macroscopic characteristics of small bowel Crohn's disease?

350 How can a Meckel's diverticulum make its owner acutely ill?

351 Besides adhesions and external hernia, what are the causes of small bowel obstruction?

352 Why is an ileostomy made the way it is?
   What is it like to have one?

The peritoneal cavity

353 How do you diagnose ascites and what are the major causes?

354 How can we treat malignant ascites?

355 What are the causes of pelvic abscess?
   How is it diagnosed and treated?

356 How do we diagnose and treat an appendix abscess?

The large bowel

357 Briefly, what is the blood supply of the large bowel?

358 What anatomical features determine that diverticular disease affects the colon, but not the rectum?

359 What structures may be damaged during mobilization of the bowel for a right hemicolectomy?

360 What are the physiological functions of the large bowel?

361 Which parts of the large bowel are most frequently affected by carcinoma?

362 How do the classical symptoms of right- and left-sided colonic cancer differ?

363 What does a rectal cancer feel like on digital examination?

364 How would you investigate an adult complaining of the passage of blood and mucus per rectum?

365 What are the operative differences between anterior resection and abdominoperineal excision of the rectum for carcinoma?
   How may the anastomosis be made in anterior resection?

366 What are the basic principles for deciding the extent of a radical operation for large bowel cancer?

367 What is the Dukes' staging system for large bowel cancer?
    What is its prognostic significance?

368 Why do we sometimes make a defunctioning colostomy at the time of an anterior resection of the rectum?
    When do we close it?

369 What large bowel conditions are premalignant?

370 What do you know about the pathophysiology of diverticular disease of the colon?

371 How common is colonic diverticular disease?

372 How does colonic diverticular disease most commonly present?

373 What advice would you give to a patient who has been shown to have uncomplicated colonic diverticular disease?

374 What are the complications of colonic diverticular disease?
    Why do they develop?

375 A man of 60 presents with a history of bleeding and mucus per rectum. Sigmoidoscopy is normal, a barium enema shows diverticular disease.
    Where do we go from here?

376 What types of rectal prolapse do you know?
    What groups develop this condition?

377 How can we treat complete rectal prolapse in an otherwise fit 70 year old?

378 What are the complications of ulcerative colitis?

379 What are the indications for surgery in ulcerative colitis?
    What are the usual surgical procedures?

380 How often does Crohn's disease affect the large bowel?
    What are its clinical manifestations?

381 What are the commonest causes of fresh bleeding per rectum?

382 Is surgery often needed for patients with brisk bleeding per rectum?
    What investigation should be carried out pre-operatively?

383 How do large bowel polyps declare themselves?

384 How do we remove colonic and rectal polyps?

The anus and anal canal

385 Which part of the anal sphincter is vital for faecal
     continence?

386 What lines the anal canal?

387 Where do piles arise within the anal canal?

388 What are the typical symptoms of piles?

389 What investigations should be carried out before we
     assume a patient's piles are the cause of his complaint
     of rectal bleeding?

390 How do we classify piles?
     How does the treatment of piles vary with their
     extent?

391 What would you do, as a surgical houseman, if a
     patient began to bleed from the operation site several
     hours after haemorrhoidectomy?

392 What is an anal fissure?
     What symptoms and signs does it produce?

393 What is a fistula-in-ano?
     How do we diagnose it?

394 How do we treat a fistula-in-ano?
     What are the dangers of operation?

395 What is the anatomy of perianal and ischiorectal
     abscess?

396 What are the principles underlying the treatment of
     perianal and ischiorectal abscess?

397 Abscesses around the anal region are sometimes
     associated with more generalized diseases.
     Can you name some?

398 What do you know of the types and mode of spread of
     cancer of the anus and anal canal?

399 What investigations should be done on a patient with
     anal warts?

400 What is a perianal haematoma and how does it
     present?

The breast

401 What is the lymphatic drainage of the breast?

402 What are the causes of a discharge from the nipple?

403 Why might a patient presenting with a breast lump also complain of increasing breathlessness?

404 What features in a breast lump might suggest that it is malignant?

405 What is the difference between skin tethering and skin fixity of a breast lump?

406 An old lady presents complaining that one breast has become much smaller than the other and the nipple replaced by a scab.
   What is the probable diagnosis?

407 What is the importance of nipple inversion?

408 What is Paget's disease of the nipple?

409 What is peau d'orange?

410 Why may the arm become swollen in breast cancer patients?

411 Does a patient with clinically obvious, apparently early breast cancer need any investigations before mastectomy?

412 Are there any advantages in pre-operative needle biopsy of a breast lump compared with excision biopsy and frozen section?

413 What is cytology?
   Can it help us in the investigation of a patient who may have breast cancer?

414 What sorts of radiological investigation help us assess a patient who may have breast cancer?

415 What is the prognostic importance of axillary lymph node involvement in a case of breast cancer?

416 What are the commonest sites of distant spread in breast cancer?

417 Do you know anything about the different theories on how breast cancer metastasizes?
   How does this problem affect our approach to treatment?

418 What do we mean by the terms 'early' and 'advanced' breast cancer in relation to treatment?

419 Who was Halsted?
   What was his contribution to the treatment of breast cancer?

420 Define 'simple' and 'radical' mastectomies.

421 What part does radiotherapy play in the treatment of early breast cancer?

422 How do we deal with the cosmetic deformity produced by mastectomy?

423 What patterns of advanced breast cancer do you know of?

424 Does surgery have any part to play in the treatment of advanced breast cancer?

425 How do bone metastases present in breast cancer?
    How do we treat them?

426 What sorts of endocrine therapy do we use in advanced breast cancer?
    How do we choose the therapy for a particular patient?

427 Why don't we leave otherwise symptomless breast lumps in young adults alone?
    Surely these aren't cancers?

428 What is a 'breast mouse'?

429 What physical signs would suggest to you that a breast lump is a simple cyst?

430 Generalized 'lumpiness' in the breasts, with or without pain, is sometimes encountered.
    What is the usual cause?

431 How may an intraduct papilloma present?

432 Do x-rays help in the investigation of a benign breast lump?

433 As a rule what is the safe course in the treatment of a breast cyst that hasn't disappeared completely on aspiration?

434 What can be done for a woman with intermittently painful breasts?

435 What is the histology of a fibro-adenoma?

436 Do you know of any benign breast disease that clinically may mimic cancer?

437 Which groups are liable to develop breast abscess?

438 What clinical features suggest breast abscess?

439 Can antibiotics cure breast infections?

440 What is the surgical treatment of a breast abscess?

441 What organisms are found in breast abscesses?

442 What is gynaecomastia?
Does it require treatment?

443 What forms of mammoplasty do you know?
What are their indications?

The endocrine system

444 How does the thyroid gland develop?
What abnormalities of development can occur?

445 How does the thyroid gland produce T3 and T4?

446 What tests can be performed to assess thyroid
function?

447 What may be the significance of a 'cold nodule' on
thyroid scanning?

448 What are the causes of a non-toxic goitre?

449 What are the histological appearances of a nodular
goitre?

450 List the possible causes of thyrotoxicosis.

451 Describe the symptoms and signs of Graves' disease.

452 How do antithyroid drugs work?
Which are used most frequently?

453 In which patients is radioactive iodine used for
treatment of thyrotoxicosis, and how effective is it?

454 What are the indications for surgery in thyrotoxicosis?

455 How is a thyrotoxic patient prepared for surgery?

456 What is the significance of an apparently solitary
thyroid nodule?

457 Why is surgery performed in patients with nodular
goitre?

458 What are the specific complications of thyroidectomy?

459 List the main types of thyroid carcinoma.

460 What is a 'lateral aberrant thyroid'?

461 Compare the clinical and histological features of
papillary and follicular carcinoma of the thyroid.

462 How does the treatment of thyroid cancer depend on
the histological type?

463 What are the various forms of thyroiditis?

464 Outline the clinical features of Hashimoto's
thyroiditis.
    How is the diagnosis confirmed and the condition
treated?

465 How do the parathyroid glands develop?
    How are they identified at operation?

466 What are the causes of hyperparathyroidism?

467 In what ways may hyperparathyroidism present?

468 How is the diagnosis of primary hyperparathyroidism
confirmed?

469 Following parathyroidectomy, hypocalcaemia may
occur.
    How is this recognised and treated?

470 What are the causes of Cushing's syndrome?

471 What are the typical features of Cushing's syndrome?

472 What is the underlying abnormality in Conn's
syndrome?
    How does this affect the patient?

473 Which patients might benefit from adrenalectomy?

474 How can a 'medical' adrenalectomy be performed?

The arteries, veins and lymphatics

475 There are two main symptoms of peripheral vascular
disease in the legs.
    What are they and what is their significance?

476 What is the natural history of intermittent
claudication?

477 Why is rest pain worse at night?

478 Outline the risk factors for the development of
atherosclerosis.

479 Atherosclerosis affects particular sites in the
peripheral vascular system.
    What are they?

480 What conditions can mimic intermittent claudication?

481 What are the major items in the examination of a
patient with peripheral vascular disease in the legs?

482 What is the significance of a femoral bruit?

483 What general advice can be given to patients with peripheral vascular disease?

484 How can peripheral vascular disease be assessed with non-invasive tests?

485 What is meant by the 'ankle/brachial pressure index', and how is it interpreted?

486 In which patients with peripheral vascular disease should aortograms be performed?

487 How are aortograms performed and what complications may occur?

488 Describe the typical pathological features of atherosclerosis.

489 Why does atheroma develop?

490 What non-operative treatment may be tried in patients with peripheral vascular disease?

491 How can a lumbar sympathectomy be performed? What does it achieve?

492 Why may diabetics get problems with their feet?

493 List the causes of acute ischaemia of the leg.

494 What are the different types of material available for arterial grafts?

495 What operations are available for the treatment of atheromatous disease in the aorto-iliac segment?

496 What are extra-anatomic grafts?

497 Where does atheroma usually affect the superficial femoral artery?

498 What is the importance of the profunda femoris artery?

499 How much does an artery need to be narrowed before there is a significant reduction in flow?

500 How may an occluded superficial femoral artery be bypassed?

501 What factors are involved with the long-term patency of grafts?

502 What are the indications for amputation in peripheral vascular disease? What principles determine the level of amputation?

503 What is an aneurysm? List the various types.

504 What is a false aneurysm? How does it develop?

505 What is an aortic dissection?

506 How may an aortic dissection present?

507 When is surgery indicated for aortic dissection?

508 How can an abdominal aortic aneurysm present?

509 Outline how a patient with an abdominal aortic aneurysm should be managed.

510 Should patients with asymptomatic aortic aneurysms have elective surgery?

511 Are all abdominal aortic aneurysms resectable?
   Are there any other methods of treatment?

512 Where can peripheral aneurysms occur?
   Who first described their surgical treatment?

513 Define an embolus and list the various types.

514 Where do peripheral arterial emboli usually lodge and what effects do they produce?

515 What does a lower limb embolectomy involve?

516 How can arteries be injured?

517 What is Buerger's disease?

518 Why may a surgeon be asked to see a case of suspected temporal arteritis urgently?

519 What is Raynaud's phenomenon?

520 In which conditions may Raynaud's phenomenon occur?

521 What is Raynaud's disease?

522 How may atheroma of the carotid artery present?

523 What is the natural history of an asymptomatic carotid bruit?

524 Outline the ways in which carotid artery atheroma can be assessed.

525 Have anti-platelet drugs been shown to be of value in carotid atheroma?

526 How is carotid surgery performed and what are the risks?

527 What is the subclavian steal syndrome?

528 How may acute mesenteric ischaemia present?

529 Ischaemic colitis produces typical radiographic
appearances.
What are they?

530 What clinical features are associated with chronic
mesenteric ischaemia?

531 What is a glomus tumour?

532 What is a carotid body tumour?

533 Do we know why varicose veins develop?

534 How would you examine a patient with varicose veins?

535 Compare the non-operative and operative treatment of
varicose veins.

536 What causes the typical features of a post-phlebitic
limb?

537 What are the physical signs of an arteriovenous fistula
in the leg and what effects can it produce?

538 What is a cystic hygroma?

Burns

539 In the assessment of the area of a burn what is the 'rule
of nines'?

540 Why is it important to assess the area and depth of
burns?

541 Why do burn patients become dehydrated?

542 How do we minimize dehydration in burn patients?

543 How may renal failure develop in burn patients?

544 How widespread must a burn be before IV fluid is
required?

545 What are the immediate steps in the management of
the badly burned patient?

546 How do we assess the fluid replacement required in a
burn patient?

547 When is blood transfusion required after a burn?

548 How do we assess the depth of a burn?

549 What parameters are monitored during the treatment
of a badly burned patient?

550 When are skin grafts required in burn patients?
Why are they used?

551 How do we prepare and apply skin grafts in the burn patient?

552 What are the major causes of death in a burn patient?

553 How do we routinely try to prevent infection of burns?

554 What are the important organisms in the infection of burns?

555 What injuries does lightning cause?

556 Which patients should be referred to specialized burns units?

557 Which burn patients are likely to suffer lung damage? How should this be managed?

Paediatric surgery

558 Should an asymptomatic inguinal hernia be operated on in the first year of life?

559 How is an irreducible inguinal hernia treated in a baby?

560 What is an umbilical hernia? How is it managed?

561 What are the surgically remediable causes of difficulty in breathing in the neonate?

562 What features suggest that a neonate has a tracheo-oesophageal fistula?

563 How may a hiatal hernia present in childhood?

564 How is hiatal hernia treated in childhood?

565 List the causes of neonatal intestinal obstruction.

566 What is the significance of bile-stained vomiting in a neonate?

567 What is meconium and when should it first be passed?

568 Why is inspection of the anus an important part of neonatal examination?

569 What are the characteristic features of congenital pyloric stenosis?

570 What is the name of the operation for this condition and what does it involve?

571 What is Hirschsprung's disease? How is it diagnosed and treated?

572 How is ileocolic intussusception treated?

573 What are the commoner causes of rectal bleeding in childhood?

574 How do we manage a child who has swallowed a safety pin?

575 What are hypospadias and epispadias?

576 What are the features of an infantile hydrocele and how is it treated?

577 Outline the possible surgical causes of neonatal obstructive jaundice.

578 What is a strawberry naevus?

579 List the commoner solid tumours of childhood.

580 How is Wilm's tumour treated?

The genito-urinary system

General points

581 What different types of pain are associated with urinary tract disease?

582 List the causes of haematuria.

583 How does the timing of haematuria in relation to micturition aid differential diagnosis?

584 If haematuria follows insignificant renal trauma what might it suggest?

585 Why is a neurological examination an essential part of a urological assessment?

586 By what criteria can a urinary infection be diagnosed in a urine sample?

587 What is sterile pyuria?
What are its main causes?

588 How is an intravenous urogram performed and what information can it provide?

589 What are the causes of calculi in the urinary tract?

590 List the types and appearances of urinary tract calculi.

591 Classify renal failure.

592 What features would suggest that renal failure might be due to obstruction in the urinary tract?

593 What is pneumaturia?
Outline its causes.

The kidney and ureter

594 Compare the physical signs of renal and splenic enlargement.

595 What simple tests of renal function are commonly used?

596 List the common congenital renal anomalies.

597 How should a space-occupying lesion in the kidney, discovered on an intravenous urogram, be assessed?

598 Why is an intravenous urogram of importance in the management of renal trauma?

599 What are the indications for surgical intervention in the management of renal trauma?

600 List the typical clinical and pathological features of acute pyelonephritis.

601 What are the commonest organisms responsible for acute pyelonephritis?

602 Outline the radiographic and pathological features of chronic pyelonephritis.

603 What are pyonephrosis and perinephric abscess?

604 What effects does tuberculosis have on the kidney and ureter?

605 How would you diagnose and treat urinary tuberculosis?

606 What are the causes of renal papillary necrosis?
     How can this present acutely?

607 Which urinary calculi are radiolucent?
     What percentage of all urinary calculi do these represent?

608 Classify renal tumours.

609 Why is 'hypernephroma' so-called?

610 What non-metastatic syndromes are associated with renal cell carcinoma?

611 How are renal tumours in adults treated?

612 What is the importance of tissue typing in renal transplantation?

613 Compare the results of cadaveric and live-related donor renal transplantation.

614 How is immunosuppression used following renal transplantation?

615 What do we mean by a duplex collecting system?

616 List the causes of bilateral hydronephrosis.

617 How is suspected pelviureteric junction obstruction diagnosed and treated?

618 How would you manage a patient with suspected ureteric colic?

619 What are the indications for surgery in ureteric calculi?

620 Define retroperitoneal fibrosis and list the causes.

621 List the commoner causes of ureteric injury.

622 What is vesico-ureteric reflux?
    How is it diagnosed?

623 How should a patient with reflux be managed?

The bladder, prostate and urethra

624 Why do patients with bladder outflow obstruction complain of frequency?

625 What are the causes of cystitis?

626 What are the appearances of the bladder in tuberculosis?

627 How does Bilharzia affect the bladder?

628 Which agents can induce malignant change in the urothelium?

629 List the common presentations of carcinoma of the bladder.

630 What types of bladder carcinoma occur?

631 How is carcinoma of the bladder diagnosed and staged?

632 How is bladder cancer treated?

633 What is an ileal conduit?

634 Why may bladder diverticula develop?
    What are their complications?

635 Define urinary incontinence and enuresis.

636 How may urodynamic studies help in the investigation of incontinence?

637 What are the principles in the management of incontinence?

638 Compare acute and chronic urinary retention.

639 List the causes of acute urinary retention.

640 How should acute post-operative retention be managed?

641 What may happen if a chronically distended bladder is decompressed too rapidly?

642 Outline the risks of prolonged catheterization.
   How may these be minimized?

643 How should patients with acute urinary retention be prepared for surgery?

644 What information about the prostate may be revealed by a rectal examination?

645 What pathological changes are found in benign prostatic hypertrophy?

646 What are the effects of prostatic enlargement on the bladder?

647 What is the significance of residual urine?

648 List the indications for prostatectomy.

649 How may prostatectomy be performed?
   What does it aim to achieve?

650 What are the complications of prostatectomy?

651 How does carcinoma of the prostate present?

652 How is the diagnosis of prostatic carcinoma proven?

653 How do we treat prostatic carcinoma?

654 What are the complications of stilboestrol therapy?

655 What are the causes of urethral stricture?

656 What are the different parts of the urethra, and which are most vulnerable to injury?

657 How does membranous urethral injury occur?
   What are its effects?

658 What is the danger in trying to pass a catheter in someone with a suspected urethral injury?

The male genitalia

659 What may cause an enlargement of the testis?

660 What do you know about the aetiology of epididymo-orchitis?

661 How do you tell the difference between acute epididymo-orchitis and testicular torsion?

662 What anatomical abnormalities are associated with testicular torsion?

663 How is a patient with suspected testicular torsion treated?

664 Classify testicular tumours.

665 How do we investigate a patient with a suspected testicular tumour?

666 How is orchidectomy performed for a testicular tumour?

667 Outline the use of radiotherapy and chemotherapy in the management of testicular tumours.

668 What is a hydrocele and what may be its cause?

669 Where does a hydrocele form in relation to the testis?

670 How can hydroceles be treated?

671 Compare the fluid from a hydrocele, spermatocele, and an epididymal cyst.

672 What is a varicocele, and what is its significance?

673 When do the testes normally reach the scrotum?

674 What do we mean by undescended, maldescended and retractile testes?

675 Where might you find a testis if it is not palpable in the scrotum?

676 What problems are associated with undescended testes?

677 When and how should undescended testes be treated?

678 What are phimosis and paraphimosis?

679 What are the common causes of impotence?

680 How is the effectiveness of vasectomy tested?

The heart, lungs and thoracic contents

681 Direct trauma may produce localized rib fractures. What problems may they cause the patient?

682 What is 'flail chest'? How would you initiate treatment?

683 When would you suspect and how would you diagnose a pneumothorax?

684 Do you understand the mechanics of a tension pneumothorax and do you know how to relieve one?

685 What are the indications for inserting a chest drain in a pneumothorax?
   Where exactly would you put it?

686 What is surgical emphysema and what does it imply?

687 How does an open chest wound impair the mechanics of breathing?
   What is the emergency management?

688 What are the considerations in positioning a patient to x-ray his injured chest?

689 If in addition to a pneumothorax your traumatized patient has fluid in the chest, how would that influence your emergency management?

690 In the hours following an accident, the driver is noted to have a widening mediastinum.
   How would you respond to this observation?

691 What are the commoner conditions that may present with haemoptysis?

692 What are the clinical and radiological features of a pleural effusion?

693 Name some diseases in which pleural effusion occurs.

694 List some of the commoner modes of presentation of lung cancer.

695 What means are now at our disposal to get a pathological diagnosis of lung cancer?

696 Where do we look for evidence of spread in a case of bronchial carcinoma?
   Why do we bother?

697 What is the differential diagnosis of mediastinal lymphadenopathy seen on a chest x-ray?

698 What are the indications for thymectomy?

699 What is an empyema and how should it be treated?

700 What is a bronchopleural fistula and when might one develop?

701 Which groups are most at risk from pulmonary tuberculosis these days?

702 What conditions can cause collapse of thoracic vertebrae?

703 Under what circumstances would you suspect fungal pulmonary infections?

704 Who are likely to inhale foreign bodies and what are the consequences?

705 Describe the clinical picture of bronchiectasis.

706 What are the indications for surgery in infective endocarditis?

707 What types of aneurysm may involve the thoracic aorta?

708 What are the lethal consequences of dissecting aneurysms affecting the ascending aorta?

709 Outline the essential components of conservative management of dissecting aneurysm of the thoracic aorta.

710 What are the neurological complications of aneurysms of the thoracic aorta?

711 Outline the possible consequences of a patent ductus arteriosus remaining unclosed into adult life.

712 Explain the clinical and chest x-ray features of coarctation of the aorta.

713 What are the four features that give Fallot's tetralogy its name?

714 What surgical management is available for rheumatic mitral valve disease?

715 Give some of the long-term complications that may be associated with cardiac valve replacement.

716 How would you recognize aortic valve stenosis clinically?

717 What are the indications for coronary artery by-pass grafting?

718 In what categories of coronary artery disease does surgery offer an improved five year survival?

719 What does angina pectoris mean literally? Do you know any other types of 'angina'?

720 Certain complications of myocardial infarction may be corrected surgically. Which are they?

721 What is involved in giving a patient a pacemaker?

Neurosurgery

722 A previously well 56 year old woman has a grand mal seizure. Clinical examination and skull x-ray are normal.
    Is further investigation required?

723 A 45 year old patient complains of severe headache, and neck stiffness is found on examination.
What points in the history help determine the cause?

724 A 60 year old man with recent weight loss of one stone, develops difficulty in walking followed by difficulty with micturition.
What is the most likely diagnosis?

725 In the above, what clinical signs would support this diagnosis?

726 Is it necessary to admit all patients with a skull fracture for observation?

727 Why must *clinical* evidence of a basal skull fracture be sought?

728 What neurological features are important in the assessment of head-injured patients?

729 What features should be observed in the assessment of level of consciousness?

730 Why is the pupil reaction to light important in head injury assessment?

731 How can limb weakness be detected in a comatose patient?

732 What radiological investigations are of most value in head injury?

733 What is the most frequently occurring type of traumatic intracranial haematoma?

734 What sites of skull fracture are associated with extradural haematoma formation?

735 Only one in two patients in coma after head injury has an intracranial haematoma.
What causes the depression of conscious level in the remainder?

736 What is the treatment of acute intracranial haematoma?

737 How do patients with chronic subdural haematoma present?

738 What operative treatment is required for chronic subdural haematoma?

739 Skull x-ray reveals a depressed fracture, underlying a deep laceration.
Is any treatment other than suture of the laceration required?

740 What are the clinical features of raised intracranial pressure?

741 How is raised intracranial pressure detected on skull x-ray?

742 If an intracranial tumour is suspected what investigations should be carried out (a) in a general hospital (b) in a neurology/neurosurgical unit?

743 What are the common types of malignant intracranial tumour?

744 If a CT scan shows an appearance typical of malignant glioma, is any further management required?

745 Which intracranial tumour can present with bilateral leg weakness?

746 Can intracranial meningiomas be removed completely at operation?
   Does incomplete removal matter?

747 What intracranial tumour is associated with von Recklinghausen's disease and how may it present?

748 How may pituitary tumours be classified?

749 What neurological deficit may be produced by pituitary tumours?

750 What are the possible routes of approach for operative removal of pituitary tumours?

751 How is the suspected diagnosis of subarachnoid haemorrhage confirmed?

752 A ruptured berry aneurysm is the commonest cause of subarachnoid haemorrhage. What are the other possible causes?

753 When a third nerve palsy presents along with clinical features of subarachnoid haemorrhage, what is the likely cause?

754 What radiological investigations are required in patients with subarachnoid haemorrhage?

755 If the patient survives the initial bleed from a ruptured aneurysm, what complications may follow?

756 What are the risks of rebleeding (a) in the first 6 months, (b) beyond the first 6 months, in a patient who has survived a ruptured berry aneurysm?

757 How can rebleeding from a berry aneurysm be prevented?

758 How may arteriovenous malformations of the brain present?

759 What features on plain spinal x-rays would suggest that cord compression is due to metastatic tumour?

760 What benign lesions cause spinal cord compression?

761 What clinical features suggest disc protrusion at the L5/S1 level?

762 What is hydrocephalus, and what are its causes?

763 How is hydrocephalus managed?

764 Who was Harvey Cushing?

Ear, nose and throat

765 How could a GP distinguish between perceptive and conductive deafness in an adult?

766 Describe exactly how you would syringe the ear.

767 How would you manage otitis externa?

768 A purulent discharge from the ear may occur with otitis media or externa. How can you tell them apart?

769 What is 'glue ear'?
    What are the causes?

770 Which organisms usually cause acute otitis media?

771 How could you distinguish between 'safe' and 'unsafe' chronic suppurative otitis media?

772 Long-standing chronic suppurative otitis media may lead to serious complications.
    What are they?

773 What is otosclerosis and how does it present?

774 What are the characteristic features of Menière's disease?

775 What is Bell's palsy and how is it managed?

776 Does tinnitus, when it is the only symptom, merit further investigation?

777 What are the typical features of presbyacusis?
    Does a hearing aid help?

778 What is the significance of cerebrospinal fluid running from the ear following a head injury?
    What would you do about it?

779 How would you deal with a patient with a broken nose?

780 What are the common causes of nose bleeds?

781 How would you treat a patient with a nose bleed?

782 List some causes of a blocked nose.

783 Are vasoconstrictor nasal sprays good or bad treatment for a blocked nose?

784 What is submucous resection of the nasal septum?

785 Allergy to dust or grass pollen is a common cause of nasal symptoms.
     What is the immunological mechanism involved?

786 What is the fundamental difference between vasomotor rhinitis and sinusitis?

787 How is sinusitis treated?

788 The prognosis for most patients with cancer of the nasal sinuses is poor.
     Why?

789 Certain diseases are associated with a membrane on the tonsils.
     What are they?

790 What are the indications for adenoidectomy?

791 How does cancer of the nasopharynx present?

792 What are the common causes of an ulcer on the tongue?

793 What is meant by a globus sensation?
     Is it an important complaint?

794 How would you diagnose a pharyngeal pouch?

795 What is meant by the Paterson-Brown-Kelly syndrome?

796 If a GP sees a patient with a hoarse voice, when should he refer him for a specialist opinion?

797 How can listening to the pattern of noisy breathing help in localizing the level of the airway obstruction?

798 What is epiglottitis?

799 A hoarse, weak voice is sometimes due to unilateral vocal cord paralysis. What are the likely causes?

800 What is the treatment for laryngeal cancer?

801 How would you deal with a patient whose only complaint was a symptomless lump in the neck?

802 What are the indications for tracheostomy?

803 What are the most important points in the immediate postoperative management of tracheostomy patients?

The eye

804 What are the signs of dysthyroid eye disease and how may vision be lost in this condition?

805 How would you examine a patient who complained of a 'floating speck' in the vision of one eye?

806 Can you name a few possible causes of unilateral proptosis in a woman of 45?

807 What is the ocular complication of oxygen therapy in premature infants?
How may it be avoided?

808 How may a cerebral tumour present to an ophthalmologist?

809 How may sarcoid affect the eye?

810 How does conjunctivitis differ from iritis in its symptomatology?

811 What are the ocular complications of herpes zoster affecting the trigeminal nerve?

812 What is a chalazion?

813 What is a dendritic ulcer?
What are the right and wrong ways of treating it?

814 The mother of a three month old child says that one of its eyes has been watering since birth.
What is the differential diagnosis?

815 What might make you think that someone had suffered a corneal abrasion?
How would you deal with it?

816 What causes of a subconjunctival haemorrhage do you know?

817 What sort of treatment should a chemical burn (acid or alkali) to the eye receive?

818 Is conjunctival pigmentation an important finding?

819 What are the symptoms of acute glaucoma?

820 What are the signs of acute glaucoma?

821 How may acute glaucoma be precipitated?

822 Can you describe the symptoms and signs of chronic simple glaucoma?

823 What are keratic precipitates?

824 Do you know how the drugs used in the management of acute glaucoma act to reduce intra-ocular pressure?

825 What circumstances may lead a casualty officer to suspect the presence of an intra-ocular foreign body?

826 Do you know any diseases which are associated with cataract formation?

827 What is aphakia?
     What are its optical disadvantages?

828 When should cataract extraction be considered?

829 What are the symptoms of optic neuritis?

830 Describe the pupil responses to light in a patient with a left optic neuritis.

831 How may papilloedema be recognized?

832 What sorts of diabetic retinopathy do you know?

833 Can diabetic retinopathy be treated?

834 What symptoms might you expect from someone with choroiditis?

835 How may a choroidal melanoma present?

836 What is night blindness and what may it signify?

837 What are the causes of sudden loss of vision in a quiet eye?

838 What is amblyopia?

839 How may drugs vary the pupil size?

840 What are the indications for squint surgery?

841 What is the significance of bitemporal hemianopic field defects to a red target?

842 What are the causes of a white pupil in a child?

Orthopaedics and fractures

Fractures: general

843 What is the difference between a simple and a compound fracture and why is the distinction an important one?

844 When can a fracture be described as 'pathological'?
Give some examples of pathological fractures.

845 Give an example of a stress fracture.

846 Describe the treatment of a compound fracture of the
tibia in the first six hours after the injury.

847 What is the principal danger of applying plaster of
Paris to a fresh fracture?
How can this danger be avoided?

848 What is meant by the term skeletal traction?
What are the common applications?

849 Fracture disease may disable the patient for months or
even years after a fracture has healed soundly and in a
good position.
What is fracture disease?

850 What is callus and what is its function?

851 How can a patient with bilateral (or even unilateral)
femoral shaft fractures die in the first few hours after
his admission to hospital, even in the absence of other
major injury?

852 Describe the clinical features of fat embolism.
What blood test is important if this condition is
suspected?

853 What factors may cause delayed or non-union of a
fracture?

854 What is Volkmann's contracture?

855 What are the degrees of peripheral nerve damage?

856 After surgical repair or an injury in continuity of a
nerve, how quickly would you expect reinnervation to
occur?

Orthopaedics: general

857 What is the commonest organism responsible for
osteomyelitis in children, and how does it reach the
bone?

858 How would you diagnose acute osteomyelitis in a
child?

859 How should acute osteomyelitis be treated?

860 Why is chronic osteomyelitis so difficult to cure?

861 Why would you be concerned about the presence of
metal or cement in the region of a bony infection?

862 How likely is it that a total hip replacement will become infected?
What can be done to minimize this risk?

863 What special hazards are there in the surgical treatment of rheumatoid arthritis?

864 What structures may be damaged by invasive rheumatoid synovium?

865 What is the classic deformity of the metacarpo-phalangeal joints in rheumatoid arthritis?

866 Describe the clinical progression of ankylosing spondylitis.
Has surgery anything to offer patients with this condition?

867 Explain the difference between osteoporosis and osteomalacia.

868 What are the main causes of osteoporosis?

869 Describe the principal features of Paget's disease of bone.

870 Describe an achondroplastic dwarf.

871 What musculoskeletal problems are encountered by a severe haemophiliac?

872 What is the commonest malignant tumour in bone?

873 Which group of patients is most at risk from osteosarcoma and what sites are most likely to develop this tumour?

874 In a young adult with an osteosarcoma of the lower end of the femur without detectable metastases, the standard treatment in the UK used to be the Cade method. Describe this treatment and the treatment more commonly used now.

875 What is osteotomy and why may it be performed?

876 What is hemiarthroplasty and what is its most common application?

877 What is meant by the term débridement?

878 What materials are commonly used in artificial joint replacements?

879 What are the commonest causes of failure of a total hip replacement?

Orthopaedics: regional

The hip and femur

880 Explain how to measure true and apparent leg length. What is the usual cause of apparent shortening?

881 What is the Trendelenburg test?
When may it be positive?

882 How do you measure fixed flexion deformity at the hip?

883 Explain why the blood supply to the head of the femur is in danger when injury occurs.

884 What structures contribute significantly to the stability of the hip joint?

885 How would you recognize clinically a fracture of the neck of the femur and why is there such a high mortality?

886 Intracapsular fractures of the neck of the femur often require replacement of the femoral head with a prosthesis.
Why?

887 Why is posterior dislocation of the hip quite easily missed?

888 Describe a central dislocation of the hip.

889 When and how should congenital dislocation of the hip be diagnosed?

890 Why is early diagnosis of CDH so important?

891 What risk factors do you know that increase the likelihood of a child's having CDH?

892 What is known of the underlying pathological process in Perthes' disease?

893 How should Perthes' disease be managed?

894 What symptoms would you expect from a child with a gradual slip of an upper femoral epiphysis?

895 What is the crucial investigation needed to make the diagnosis of slipped upper femoral epiphysis?

896 What operations, other than total hip replacement, are available for primary osteo-arthritis of the hip joint?

897 Describe the main contra-indications to total hip replacement.

898 How would you recognize a septic arthritis of the hip?

899 Describe the typical radiological appearances of rheumatoid arthritis in the hip.

900 Assuming that other major injuries have been excluded, what is the emergency treatment of a fractured shaft of the femur?

901 Describe the use of a Thomas' splint.

The knee and lower leg

902 What are the functions of the menisci?

903 What is the normal angle of the femur on the tibia?

904 What is meant by a 'locked' knee and what are the usual causes?

905 How do you test for medial or lateral collateral ligament laxity?

906 What changes would you expect in the rest of the limb after any derangement of the knee?

907 In an injured knee what is the significance of tenderness above the joint line as opposed to at the joint line?

908 What investigations other than plain radiography might be used to investigate an injured knee?

909 Where is the commonest site for a meniscus to tear?

910 What is the likely course of events in the years following meniscectomy?

911 Why may it be difficult to distinguish an acute complete ligament tear from a partial tear or strain?
    Why is this important?

912 What is osteochondritis dissecans of the knee, and how does it present?

913 What do we mean by an unstable patella and how can it be treated?

914 What is genu varum?
    Why is this deformity likely to give trouble?

915 What operations can be offered to a patient with severe rheumatoid arthritis of the knee?

916 What is the important difference between a displaced and an undisplaced fracture of the patella?

917 What pathological process occurs in Osgood-Schlatter's disease?

918 What is the commonest method of treating closed fractures of the tibia?

919 Describe external skeletal fixation of a fractured tibia.
     What are its advantages?

The ankle and foot

920 What damage is done in the common 'sprained ankle'?

921 Why is it important to get anatomical reduction in
     fractures involving the ankle joint?

922 What is the difference between a bunion and hallux
     valgus?

923 What is hallux rigidus?

924 What is metatarsalgia?

925 What is the other name for club foot?
     Describe the deformity.

926 Do flat feet commonly cause symptoms?

The spine

927 What are the consequences of bilateral sacral root
     damage due to central disc prolapse?

928 Why do displaced fractures and dislocations occur more
     commonly in the cervical and lumbar regions than in
     the thoracic spine?

929 Outline the structure of an intervertebral disc.

930 A surprising degree of structural scoliosis may be
     missed on inspection of the back. What is the best
     method of demonstrating the deformity?

931 What is the significance of limitation of straight leg
     raising?

932 What physical signs would you look for in a patient
     with spondylolisthesis?

933 What is the significance of feeling a soft, yielding area
     between the spinous processes of two vertebrae
     following trauma?

934 Where may a psoas abscess become palpable?
     What is the other major physical sign in this
     condition?

935 What is a myelogram?

936 What lesion is shown by oblique x-ray of the lumbar
     spine?

937 All patients who have been hit on the head and
     concussed should have a radiograph of the cervical
     spine. Where are serious injuries most commonly
     missed?

938 How are the majority of disc prolapses treated?

939 When is prolapsed lumbar intervertebral disc a surgical emergency?

940 What is the difference between 'laminectomy' and 'disc excision'?

941 Define spondylolisthesis, spondylolysis and spondylosis.

942 What can be done surgically for a spondylolisthesis of L5 on S1?

943 In developed countries, what is the commonest and most disabling form of scoliosis?

944 How should a patient with a suspected unstable injury of the thoracolumbar spine be nursed?

945 Why is it important that a patient with rheumatoid arthritis should have a neck x-ray before having an operation?

946 What is the usual treatment for an unstable injury of the cervical spine?

947 What were the main causes of death in patients with spinal cord injuries before the development of special centres for treatment?

The shoulder and arm

948 What are the clinical features of anterior dislocation of the shoulder?

949 What proportion of abduction of the shoulder is scapulothoracic and what proportion takes place at the glenohumeral joint?

950 What structures form the rotator cuff and what is its function?

951 Describe the course of the circumflex nerve.
     Why is this clinically important?

952 What views may be obtained in addition to the plain PA and lateral films when investigating the shoulder joint?

953 Why is posterior dislocation of the shoulder easily missed?

954 How do you reduce an anterior dislocation of the shoulder?

955 Explain the mechanism behind recurrent dislocation of the shoulder. What can be done surgically to treat it?

956 How would you treat a fractured clavicle in a young adult?

957 Sir Robert Peel, a Prime Minister in the nineteenth century and founder of the Metropolitan Police, died of a fractured clavicle.
Why did this kill him?

958 Which injuries of the upper limb require treatment with a collar-and-cuff sling rather than a long arm sling?

959 What is a 'frozen shoulder' in pathological terms?

960 Describe the painful arc syndrome.

961 What can be done for the severely damaged rheumatoid shoulder which is giving a lot of pain?

962 Describe a Colles' fracture.

963 How would you treat a Colles' fracture in an old lady?

964 Describe a Monteggia fracture-dislocation.

965 What is the principal danger of supracondylar fracture of the humerus in children?

The hand

966 How can you test the function of the deep and superficial flexor tendons to the fingers?

967 What is the usual sensory innervation of the hand?

968 What signs would you expect in a hand with chronic loss of median innervation?

969 What would you expect to find in a hand without ulnar innervation?

970 What is the only small muscle of the hand consistently innervated by the median nerve and how do you test it?

971 What is the main deficit if the radial nerve is divided above the elbow?

972 What types of grip do you know?

973 What is the blood supply of the scaphoid bone?

974 What is trigger finger?

975 The hand can get stiff very easily when injured. What can be done to avoid the oedema that leads to stiffness?

976 Which is more important to the function of the hand, muscle power or sensation?

977 Describe the diagnosis and treatment of a fractured scaphoid.

978 How can stable fractures of the phalanges be treated?

979 What is Bennett's fracture of the thumb?

980 What is often described as 'no man's land' in flexor
     tendon injuries?

981 What should a casualty officer do if he suspects a cut
     flexor tendon at the level of the proximal phalanx?

982 Why are infections liable to cause a great deal of
     damage to a hand?

983 What is the correct treatment if pus is suspected in a
     hand?

984 In general terms, how should superficial burns
     involving the hand be managed?

985 Describe a grease-gun injury to the hand.

986 What is the significance of a human bite injury over
     the metacarpophalangeal joint?

987 What are the classical symptoms and signs of
     compression of the median nerve in the carpal
     tunnel?

988 What is de Quervain's syndrome?

989 What is the clinical picture in Dupuytren's disease of
     the hand?

990 What is a ganglion?

What is . . .?

991 What is a cyst?

992 What is a fistula?

993 What is a sinus?

994 What is an ulcer?

995 What is a carbuncle?

996 What is an empyema?

997 What is a felon?

998 What is Courvoisier's Law?

999 What is Sister Marie-Joseph's nodule?

1000 Who was Gazornenplat?

2 Answers

'On the spot'

1 From the story and findings one can assume a major intra-abdominal event has given rise to peritonitis. While considering the differential diagnosis, I would put up a drip and arrange investigations before proceeding to appropriate treatment. The differential diagnosis is primarily between a perforated peptic ulcer and acute pancreatitis. Investigations required are full blood count, urea and electrolytes, serum amylase, group and save serum, erect and supine abdominal films, erect chest x-ray, and an ECG. In the absence of free gas on the x-ray, and amylase over 1000 would suggest pancreatitis. If free gas is noted, however, or if the amylase level is non-diagnostic, operation is indicated.

2 Blood dripping from the nose or mouth is a certain sign of postoperative haemorrhage. If no blood is visible, excessive swallowing is suggestive that bleeding is continuing and the breathing may be noisy as the blood bubbles in the pharynx. Swallowed blood is very irritant to the stomach and a sudden vomit of fresh blood is an indication of significant haemorrhage. Later, there will be signs of shock with tachycardia, hypotension, pallor, sweating and restlessness. By this time, there is a serious threat to life.

3 In view of the recent cardiac history, this clinical picture is highly suggestive of mesenteric infarction due to embolism of a mural thrombus formed on the infarcted myocardium. Other coincidental abdominal emergencies are possible, but much less likely.

4 The diagnosis of temporal arteritis should be suspected and this may be supported by a grossly raised ESR. Urgent temporal artery biopsy should be performed although therapy should not necessarily be delayed until the result is available. Treatment consists of high doses of prednisolone in order to control the arteritis rapidly and to prevent contralateral ophthalmic artery occlusion which would result in total blindness.

5 Very little. A penny will pass through the alimentary tract of a two year old without difficulty. The mother should be strongly reassured, but perhaps told to watch out for the coin in the child's stool. It can be expected to have passed by the sixth day.

6 If leaking aortic aneurysm is strongly suspected but unconfirmed, rapid preparations should be made for laparotomy, including the cross-match of 10 units of blood, at the same time carrying out quickly several important investigations. An ECG should be done to exclude myocardial infarction, although the pain would be unusual for this diagnosis. Chest x-ray and abdominal films including a 'lateral abdominal shoot-through' will allow a search for aortic calcification which may delineate an aneurysm. Abdominal ultrasound, if rapidly available, is also useful in the confirmation of an aneurysm. Finally, a serum amylase should be done quickly to exclude pancreatitis. If a non-surgical cause of the presentation is not found then laparotomy should be performed with urgency.

7 He presents the clinical picture of Boerhaave's syndrome, and has suffered a rupture of the thoracic oesophagus, due to very high intra-oesophageal pressure caused by vomiting. The surgeons will arrange a chest x-ray to confirm rupture into the left pleura, as is usual, and perhaps place a chest drain to relieve any cardiorespiratory embarrassment produced by the leak. The most important step is preparation for urgent thoracotomy to clean out the affected pleural cavity, debride the oesophageal tear, and lay open the mediastinal pleura to minimize chemical and bacterial mediastinitis. Two large chest drains will be inserted prior to closure. Broad spectrum antibiotics will be prescribed, and a feeding gastrostomy or jejunostomy made, so that the oesophagus is temporarily bypassed.

8 This patient is exhibiting Charcot's triad, that is jaundice, right upper abdominal pain, and fever, suggesting that she has acute obstructive cholangitis. This is a very serious condition, demanding rapid recognition and treatment.

9 The most likely causes of haematemesis in this young alcoholic are oesophageal varices and peptic ulcer, while others include erosive gastritis and a Mallory-Weiss tear. Management depends to a large extent on precise diagnosis, so, when resuscitation has been carried out, upper GI endoscopy is required to make the differential diagnosis.

10 The story suggests that the patient has renal colic, so early management includes symptomatic relief, and examination and investigation to establish the diagnosis and define the cause. He should be given adequate analgesia, always bearing in mind the possibility that the patient may be a pethidine addict in search of a 'fix'. A history of previous episodes, recent trauma or the symptoms of disordered calcium metabolism should be sought. The urine should be inspected visually, tested for blood and protein, sent for culture, and sieved for stones. An IVU is carried out soon after admission and blood taken for calcium estimation.

11 The clinical picture suggests two main possibilities, both causing diaphragmatic irritation—these are a sub-phrenic abscess and left lower lobe pneumonia. After physical examination, a chest x-ray is taken to look for signs of these lesions. However, this may not be conclusive as pneumonic changes can develop secondary to subphrenic abscess, and an elevated diaphragm can occur with pulmonary collapse/consolidation. Therefore further investigations are required, usually ultrasonography, or x-ray screening of the diaphragm for paradoxical movement.

12 The most likely cause of her problem is inflammatory bowel disease, usually ulcerative colitis. Other possibilities include infective lesions, especially amoebiasis if she has been abroad, while *Salmonella* and *Shigella* are less likely to cause bleeding. Although very unlikely at this age, carcinoma should not be forgotten. Stool should be sent for microscopy and culture, and sigmoidoscopy and mucosal biopsy performed. So long as perforation or toxic megacolon are not suspected (in which case plain abdominal films are ordered) an instant enema (a barium examination without preparation) is carried out looking mainly for evidence of inflammatory bowel disease.

13 The story of vomiting so much blood is usually exaggerated by a frightened patient or relative. Nevertheless, it sounds as though a significant bleed has occurred, and it must be assessed with urgency. If the patient shows obvious signs of haemorrhage, it is best to put up a drip, arrange baseline blood tests and cross-match four to six pints of blood at the outset. Next, a history and examination may reveal use of ulcerogenic drugs in view of his arthritis, in which case a peptic ulcer or gastric erosions should be suspected. In this age group carcinoma of the stomach is also a possibility. After adequate resuscitation, upper GI endoscopy should be performed to define the source of

the bleed. Further management involves careful monitoring and blood replacement; gastric erosions usually respond to conservative therapy, while if the diagnosis is peptic ulcer, surgery will be required for major continuing or repeated haemorrhage.

14 No. A major intraperitoneal haemorrhage is in progress and requires urgent laparotomy if exsanguination is to be avoided. Careful anaesthesia should not influence the outcome of the head injury. If the patient simultaneously shows evidence of an intracranial haemorrhage, then exploration of the head and abdomen can be performed simultaneously.

15 The most likely cause of this patient's breathlessness is a pneumothorax which has progressively enlarged and is now under tension. The original minor accident may have caused one or more rib fractures with injury to the lung, leading to progressive accumulation of air; the presence of surgical emphysema would confirm this suspicion. Increased resonance and reduced or absent breath sounds on the side of the lesion will be found, and deviation of the trachea and displacement of the apex beat would support the diagnosis of tension. Whenever possible, a chest x-ray should be seen before an attempt is made to treat pneumothorax, but in an emergency the tension should be relieved by inserting an IV cannula between the ribs. If the diagnosis is correct, air will rush out with an audible hiss and the patient's distress will be relieved rapidly.

16 The history strongly suggests recurrent transient ischaemic episodes, which are usually due to small emboli shed from atheromatous ulcers in the extracranial carotid arteries. Petit mal fits are the other possibility. If there is a history or signs of atheromatous disease, especially if a carotid bruit is present, the doctor must refer the patient urgently for a vascular opinion, as early carotid surgery may prevent a dense stroke or even death.

17 All the features of this story suggest a diagnosis of intussusception, a condition seen in weaning babies in which one part of the bowel, usually the distal ileum, telescopes into the lumen distal to it, possibly due to the action of peristalsis on hypertrophied mucosal lymphoid tissue. The diagnosis can often be made on the history and examination, but x-rays, including barium enema, may be required to confirm it. Examination may reveal a mass, usually in the upper abdomen. Rectal examination occasionally detects the head of the intussusception in the rectum; on withdrawal of the finger, bloody mucus will be found on the glove in most cases. Plain x-ray will show small bowel obstruction, while a barium enema will produce

the typical 'coiled spring' pattern as the contrast spreads between the head of the intussusception and the surrounding bowel wall.

18 He has almost certainly developed a pseudocyst of the pancreas. In this condition the lesser sac fills with an exudate consisting mainly of pancreatic secretion, surrounded by a layer of acute inflammatory tissue. The best way to confirm the diagnosis is by ultrasonography; lateral barium studies will show a mass pushing the stomach forwards.

19 This man has almost certainly suffered a pelvic fracture which has caused injury to his membranous urethra. Catheterization, especially by someone like me, is liable to induce further damage to the urethra, so I would leave his further urological assessment to the urologists—while they were coming, I would examine the patient carefully to exclude any other important injuries.

20 Having checked that the patient does not require immediate resuscitation, the cause of the bleed should be sought. Sometimes such a bleed is due simply to piles, but a large haemorrhage in a patient in whom there is blood in the rectum without an obvious anal lesion is most likely to be bleeding from diverticular disease or angiodysplasia. In both conditions the blood is usually dark. Haemorrhage stops spontaneously in at least 80 per cent, so that bed rest and blood replacement are all that are required in the short term. If haemorrhage continues, selective angiography is the best way to site the bleeding—barium studies and colonoscopy are usually unhelpful. Radiographic detection of one of these lesions in a patient who continues to bleed is an indication for emergency resection.

21 This syndrome is highly suggestive of saddle embolism in a patient with atrial fibrillation; having formed a clot in the left atrium due to her fibrillation, part of the clot has escaped, to lodge at the bifurcation of the aorta. Clinical examination and an ECG will confirm the dysrhythmia, while the findings of absent pulses in cold, pale, weak legs in which sensory changes are appearing distally will confirm the vascular occlusion.

22 The most likely cause of this clinical picture is carcinoma of the oesophagus or cardia, although there are other possibilities; dysphagia for solids but not liquids suggests a mechanical hold-up, so a benign stricture could be present, but this is unlikely without a history of heartburn due to hiatus hernia. Occasionally this picture can result from compression

of the oesophagus by a mediastinal mass, such as advanced bronchial carcinoma. Investigation will include a barium swallow to confirm a mechanical lesion and show its outline (a carcinoma will show as an irregular stricture of variable length, perhaps with shouldering), and endoscopy which will allow direct visualization and biopsy.

23 I think I would try to allay her fears by telling her that breast cancer does not usually produce local pain, so that this diagnosis is not top of the list of possibilities. I would look for a history of cyclical pain and would examine the breasts and axillae carefully. If the lump was smooth, spherical and firm, especially with a cyclical history of pain, I would attempt aspiration. If fluid were found and the lump disappeared after aspiration I would send her home greatly relieved, but would check her again in six weeks. This would be the most likely course of events. However, if aspiration were unsuccessful, I would arrange biopsy excision.

24 All the clinical features point towards a diagnosis of ischaemic colitis. This condition is commonest in people with pre-existing atheromatous disease. Pathologically, it consists of an ischaemic lesion, usually involving the splenic flexure of the colon, affecting the mucosa primarily. In most cases the symptoms resolve on conservative measures.

25 She is exhibiting the typical features of the carcinoid syndrome, which occurs in patients in whom a carcinoid tumour, or argentaffinoma, usually of small bowel origin, has metastasized to the liver. Her abdominal pain and diarrhoea are likely to be due to the stimulatory effect on the bowel of 5-hydroxytryptamine, released by the tumour, though the pain may sometimes indicate obstruction due to the primary lesion. Facial flushing is due to cutaneous vasodilatation, while the shortness of breath may be secondary to bronchiolar construction, both due to high circulating levels of 5H-T.

26 The unconscious patient who has been the subject of major trauma needs careful but rapid assessment of all systems in a particular order of priority. Great care must be taken if there is any suspicion of a spinal injury particularly in the cervical region. Immediately, the airway must be checked and cleared; difficulty with ventilation, either due to upper airway damage or chest injury, may require the passage of an endotracheal tube, especially as hypoxia causes brain swelling, exacerbating the head injury. At the same time major external haemorrhage must be stopped. Major thoracic injuries, producing pneumo- or

haemothorax, must be recognized and dealt with next. The abdomen is then examined, looking for evidence of 'run-over' injury and intraperitoneal haemorrhage, using lavage if uncertain. All the above types of injury carry an immediate threat to life. What remains are the medium-term problems, including assessment of the head injury—perhaps including the giving of dexamethasone to reduce cerebral oedema—a check for pelvic and urological injuries, and finally limb injuries.

27 It sounds very much as though he has developed gas gangrene, either due to simple inoculation of the organism into a dirty wound, or as an endogenous infection due to perforation of the rectum by the spike. There are four things to do to save his life: first, he must be started on large doses of penicillin to try to confine the Clostridial infection; second, an EUA is necessary to decide if the bowel has been damaged—pre-operative x-rays will also help—and if this has occurred a proximal colostomy is required; third, the buttock wound must be carefully debrided, to remove dead and dirty tissue; finally, treatment in a hyperbaric oxygen chamber is required to eradicate the Clostridial infection.

28 He is suffering from intermittent swelling of a submandibular salivary gland, probably due to a stone in Wharton's duct.

The acute abdomen

General clinical features

29 The cardinal features of such a pain are its constancy, and the fact that it is made worse by movement. The constancy contrasts with the intermittent pain caused by the muscular contraction of an obstructed viscus. The movements which exacerbate this pain may include those due to breathing, coughing, yawning or movement of the whole body, as in turning over in bed—hence the patient tends to lie very still.

30 This is the convenient term applied to a syndrome produced by an intra-abdominal inflammatory lesion causing peritoneal inflammation. A patient is said to exhibit peritonism when he complains of a constant abdominal pain, which is worse on movement, and in whom guarding and rebound tenderness may be demonstrable. Thus, peritonism is present in such conditions as appendicitis, cholecystitis, ruptured ectopic pregnancy, and perforated duodenal ulcer, but does not automatically suggest the presence of free,

abnormal peritoneal fluid, implicit in the conventional use of the more sinister term peritonitis.

31   Yes. The patient with irritation of the diaphragmatic peritoneum will often complain of shoulder tip pain because the diaphragm receives its nerve supply via C4 in the phrenic nerve. The diaphragmatic irritation may be due to subphrenic abscess, free gut content, as in perforated ulcer, or free blood due to a ruptured spleen or ectopic pregnancy. Similarly, referred pain in the area of the scapula may occur in cholecystitis.

32   These are abdominal colic, distension, vomiting and constipation. The precise order in which the symptoms occur helps determine the anatomical level of the obstruction.

33   While 'faecal' vomiting indicates the actual vomiting of faeces, the term 'faeculent' means that the vomitus merely simulates faeces. Faeculent vomiting occurs in established small bowel obstruction—the vomitus becomes brown and offensive due to the heavy overgrowth of bowel organisms. This relatively common finding must be distinguished from the rare faecal vomiting which follows gastrocolic fistula due to benign peptic ulcer, or cancer of the stomach or colon.

34   While guarding is a reliable sign of significant intra-abdominal pathology, tenderness is less so. The presence of tenderness is a subjective sign, requiring palpation followed by the patient's interpretation of what it felt like. While intra-abdominal lesions such as appendicitis and cholecystitis, will certainly induce tenderness, this sign may also be found in patients with non-specific 'tummy upsets', or even in the nervous patient without demonstrable pathology. Guarding, on the other hand, is a more objective physical sign. It is similarly demonstrated by gentle abdominal palpation, and is produced by a sustained reflex increase in the resting tone of the abdominal wall muscles, either locally or generally, in response to parietal peritoneal inflammation of whatever cause. It should be carefully distinguished from the sudden increase in tone produced by the clumsy examining hand, confusingly known as 'voluntary guarding'.

35   One is looking for signs of peritoneal inflammation, distension, visible peristalsis and localized masses, including external herniae. Peritoneal inflammation may lead to a decrease in the normal abdominal wall movement produced by breathing. In generalized peritonitis such movement disappears completely. If respiratory movement remains, the patient should be asked to distend and retract the abdomen voluntarily.

This is usually painful and reduced in patients with parietal peritoneal inflammation. If the examiner is still unsure, the patient can be asked to cough, gently at first, then more forcibly if necessary—this will produce pain in the presence of an inflammatory lesion—the patient may hesitate or even refuse to cough, a useful pointer to significant pathology. The presence of distension is sometimes difficult to decide upon, as abdominal shape is so variable between subjects. It is worth asking the patient or relatives if the abdomen is enlarged in equivocal cases.

36 The most common, and hence most important, conditions which can cause acute abdominal symptoms are pneumonia and cardiac disease, either failure or infarction. Another very important group are childhood acute viral illnesses. Pneumonia, especially involving the bases, can produce marked abdominal pain, with tenderness and guarding, while acute cardiac disease, perhaps due to hepatic engorgement, can cause a similar picture. Upper respiratory tract infections in children are sometimes accompanied, or even masked, by an abdominal syndrome mimicking appendicitis. Careful questioning will usually elicit the relevant non-abdominal symptoms. Other less common problems are raised by herpes zoster, diabetes, and very rarely porphyria and syphilis.

37 Central back pain, usually accompanied by other characteristic symptoms and signs, is often present in cases of acute pancreatitis, and in leaking aortic aneurysm. Central pain may also be present in those with an acute exacerbation of gastric or duodenal ulcer symptoms, in whom the ulcer is penetrating the posterior wall to involve the pancreas. Lateral back pain, particularly in the loin, may be due to renal or ureteric disease, usually a stone. Higher on the right, such pain may indicate acute cholecystitis or biliary colic.

38 'Rebound tenderness' refers to the pain produced by sudden, deliberate movement of the abdominal wall in cases of intra-abdominal inflammation. It is due to involvement of the parietal peritoneum in the inflammatory process, and can be induced by the examiner by various manoeuvres aimed at causing sudden friction between the parietal peritoneum and the abdominal contents. The conventional technique to elicit the sign involves carefully applying pressure at a point, for instance the right iliac fossa, followed by sudden release of the examining hand. This is normally painless but is very painful in the presence of disease. It is important to warn the patient of the impending test as their surprised gasp caused by the

sudden movement may be mistaken for a positive test. This technique is rather unkind; a more civilized manoeuvre requires simple percussion of the abdomen, producing a lesser, more controlled, excursion of the abdominal wall.

Appendicitis

39 In pathological terms, appendicitis usually develops secondary to obstruction of the appendiceal lumen, leading to infection of the pent-up mucus. In children this may be due simply to hypertrophy of a lymphoid follicle in the wall of the appendix, while in adults a faecalith is the more common cause. Unusually, appendicitis follows luminal obstruction due to caecal carcinoma, Crohn's disease or the presence of fruit seeds or intestinal worms.

40 The first symptom in this condition is usually central abdominal pain. Soon afterwards anorexia and malaise develop, while the pain moves within a few hours to the right iliac fossa, where it is constant and worse with movement. Vomiting may occur in unspectacular amounts, while the bowel habit may be unchanged, constipated or somewhat loose. On examination, the patient usually looks listless and may be flushed. The tongue is dirty and the temperature usually raised no higher than 38°C. Unless perforation has occurred, breathing movements of the abdomen are present but palpation reveals tenderness, guarding and rebound tenderness. Rovsing's sign (RIF pain following the rebound test in the LIF) is a reliable sign. Rectal examination is required only if the diagnosis is not obvious after abdominal examination; pelvic appendicitis is best confirmed this way.

41 The appendix, like the rest of the bowel, is innervated solely by the autonomic system. Intestinal autonomic pain is poorly localized, and felt in the midline. As with the rest of the mid-gut, appendiceal pain occurs around the umbilicus. As the condition progresses, the inflammatory process spreads through the wall of the appendix to involve the parietal peritoneum. This excites the somatic nerves supplying the abdominal wall, enabling the patient to locate the pathology accurately to the right iliac fossa.

42 This point lies at the junction of the lateral third and medial two-thirds of a line joining the right anterior superior iliac spine and the umbilicus. It has three important uses, anatomical, clinical and operative. Anatomically it roughly indicates the surface marking of the base of the appendix, clinically it is usually the site of maximal tenderness in appendicitis, while at

operation it marks the midpoint of the classical McBurney's incision for appendicectomy.

43 He would probably survive. In most cases the omentum would wrap itself around the appendix, preventing progression to spreading peritonitis should the appendix rupture. Within this inflammatory mass, the episode might resolve by simple 'burning out' of the inflammatory process. The appendix would be left scarred and distorted, and liable to recurrent episodes. Alternatively an abscess might form in the mass; this serious event would probably resolve by spontaneous drainage of the abscess into the rectum, colon or through the skin. In some cases, however, the omentum would fail to localize the condition, so that perforation would lead to generalized peritonitis, septicaemia, renal failure, hepatic sepsis and the death of the patient.

44 The most likely explanation is that the patient has developed an appendix mass. This usually develops in a case not treated within four or five days of the onset of symptoms. The omentum has become wrapped around the appendix, producing a phlegmon, or simple inflammatory mass. Operation is avoided, as appendicectomy would be difficult and hazardous due to the danger of damaging the bowel around the mass. However, should the temperature begin to swing, suggesting an abscess had developed, or if signs of spreading peritonitis appear, surgery is required. Less likely, but very important causes of an RIF mass in a patient with suspected appendicitis are Crohn's disease, or a caecal carcinoma which is obstructing the appendix.

45 It must be assumed that an infection is present and the site looked for. In the first few postoperative days, a chest infection is the most likely explanation. Wound infection, heralded by local pain, tenderness and erythema, usually presents around the fourth to seventh day. Intra-abdominal sepsis is less common; a pelvic abscess, suggested by pelvic discomfort and diarrhoea, is diagnosed in rectal examination. Urinary infection and deep vein thrombosis should be excluded.

46 He should exclude several possible inflammatory lesions, notably Meckel's diverticulitis, acute salpingitis, cholecystitis and terminal ileal Crohn's disease. Free fluid in the peritoneal cavity will give a clue to several other conditions—gastric content will suggest a perforated peptic ulcer, which can sometimes mimic appendicitis, while free blood will usually be due to a ruptured ectopic pregnancy or a twisted ovarian cyst.

Biliary disease

47 The illness begins with worsening epigastric and right subcostal pain, which becomes severe, constant and worse during inspiration. The pain may radiate to the right scapular region. Nausea and vomiting are variable. On examination the patient, usually female and often obese, will have a moderate pyrexia. Occasionally a fleeting jaundice will be noted. Tenderness and guarding will be found mainly in the right subcostal region. Murphy's sign (reflex inhibition of inspiration when the examining hand is pressed under the costal margin) is often present.

48 Yes. The remarkable feature was the severity of the pain. The patient had developed right upper quadrant pain a few hours before; the pain was agonizing and had not been intermittent, like intestinal colic. She retched violently several times. Although she was in a cold sweat, the temperature was normal. The gall bladder was palpable, and fairly tender. The pain was greatly relieved by an injection of pethidine, and did not return when the pethidine wore off.

49 Yes. Ultrasonography and HIDA-radio-isotope scanning can both be used. Ultrasonography can confirm the presence of gall-stones, demonstrate the thickened wall of the gall bladder, and determine whether it is distended. HIDA-scanning involves injecting an isotope-labelled substance which is rapidly excreted in the bile. In acute cholecystitis, the obstructed gall bladder will not admit the labelled bile, and therefore will not be visualized on a scan. Clinical diagnosis alone is wrong in 10 to 15 per cent of cases of acute cholecystitis, so these tests are particularly useful if surgery is practised routinely in the acute phase.

50 Most surgeons treat acute cholecystitis conservatively. The aim is to 'rest' the gall bladder in the knowledge that the episode will settle within a week without complications in 85 per cent of patients. As gall bladder contraction is stimulated by cholecystokinin, released from the duodenum when chyme enters it, gall bladder 'rest' requires cessation of oral intake, and hence intravenous fluids.

51 This is a rather controversial question. Some surgeons believe that all patients with this diagnosis should undergo cholecystectomy at the next elective operating list, arguing that this halves the period of hospitalization, and that urgent surgery does not increase mortality, morbidity or difficulty of operation. Most surgeons have yet to adopt this policy; their

indications are therefore much more limited, involving only the 15 per cent of patients who go on to develop empyema or gangrene of the gall bladder, or biliary peritonitis, all diagnosed by careful clinical monitoring during conservative management.

52 Yes, it can be lethal, especially if treatment is delayed. Usually it is due to duct obstruction by gall-stones. Organisms multiply in the obstructed duct leading to septicaemia. The classical Charcot's triad of jaundice, pain and fever gives the diagnosis, and biliary ultrasonography can confirm the underlying problem. After taking blood cultures, broad spectrum antibiotics, for instance, gentamicin, ampicillin and metranidazole, are given. Urine output is monitored using a catheter, and septic shock dealt with. Drainage of the biliary tree, akin to the drainage of an abscess, is required urgently if there has not been a dramatic improvement within 12 to 24 hours. This will require laparotomy, duct exploration and placement of a T-tube. Recently, however, endoscopic sphincterotomy and stone removal has become available and may be much safer in the very ill patient.

53 This is the name given to small bowel obstruction due to a gallstone. It is an uncommon condition—two per cent of all cases of intestinal obstruction—occurring mainly in elderly females. Almost always the stone enters the small bowel via a cholecyst-duodenal fistula. The clinical picture is of typical small bowel obstruction which may be intermittent as the stone moves on. X-rays may show gas in the biliary tree, small bowel fluid levels, an opaque stone away from the gall bladder, or the disappearance from the gall bladder of a stone noted at a previous examination. The diagnosis is often delayed, and the mortality remains at about five to ten per cent.

Perforated peptic ulcer

54 Perforated duodenal ulcers are fairly uniform in appearance—almost always the perforation is circular, about three to five mm in diameter, and looks so neat that it might have been made with a ticket-punch. Occasionally a piece of undigested food will be seen impacted in the perforation. The duodenal wall around the defect is usually stiff and friable due to oedema. The site of perforation in over 90 per cent of cases is the middle of the anterior wall of the first part of the duodenum.

55 Yes, it certainly can differ. The great majority of patients with this condition present with the classical story of sudden onset of agonizing epigastric pain which

rapidly becomes generalized. On examination the patient lies still, afraid to move for fear of the pain, appears shocked, and has a rigid, silent abdomen. In the elderly, however, although the classical picture is often seen, some present in a much less dramatic way. The pain may be mild, and the abdomen tender but not rigid. It is easy to underestimate the problem. Absent bowel sounds are a major clue, and the blood pressure may be unexpectedly low. The rule is always to be wary of any abdominal symptoms or signs in the elderly.

56 The erect chest x-ray. The cardinal radiological sign is free gas under the diaphragm, and this can be missed on the erect abdominal film. The reason for this is that the x-ray exposure necessary to penetrate the abdomen is greater than that for the chest. Thus, even though the diaphragm may be included in the erect abdominal film, it may not be visible due to the high x-ray exposure, so that subphrenic gas will appear in continuity with the lung, and hence be missed. The chest x-ray, however, exposed so as to show fine lung detail, will demonstrate the diaphragm with gas below and lung above. Nevertheless in 30 per cent of perforations gas is not present under the diaphragm.

57 Yes, always a serum amylase and often an ECG. All the symptoms and signs of perforated ulcer can, and often do, occur in acute pancreatitis. Myocardial infarction can sometimes present as an 'abdominal catastrophe', so this possibility must be excluded if doubt exists. Basal pneumonia will already have been excluded by the routine erect chest x-ray. Having taken these precautions, laparotomy is mandatory despite the lack of free gas on x-ray, as the latter is not seen in 30 per cent of perforations, while other conditions which can mimic perforated ulcer, such as mesenteric infarction and leaking aneurysm, all require operative management.

58 The usual operations are simple oversew for duodenal ulcer and partial gastrectomy for gastric ulcer. Oversew in duodenal ulcer is most surgeons' choice as it is quick and safe, the ulcer is never malignant, and 25 per cent will never have any further ulcer symptoms. However, some surgeons believe more definitive ulcer surgery, usually vagotomy, should be performed, especially in those with a history of dyspepsia. Simple oversew is never enough in gastric ulcer—10 per cent of these are malignant, and the ulcer is often large and ragged, making closure impossible or unsafe. Most surgeons, therefore, would do a Billroth I gastrectomy, while

others would excise the ulcer to exclude malignancy and perform a vagotomy.

59   There is no doubt that surgery offers the best chance for survival if the patient can withstand the operation. Therefore, the assistance and advice of a senior anaesthetist and a physician where indicated, should be urgently sought with the aim of improving the general condition sufficiently to allow surgery. With non-operative management several outcomes are possible. The ulcer may seal and the condition gradually settle, the free gastric fluid may lead to a localized abscess such as a subphrenic, or septicaemia and death may supervene. Management should therefore include meticulous nasogastric suction to minimize leakage, careful fluid balance, broad spectrum antibiotics to cover the expected septicaemia, and a watch for abscess formation. The patient is best nursed semi-erect so that any abscess formation is pelvic rather than subphrenic. This position will also aid breathing in these sick patients.

60   Corticosteroids, aspirin, phenylbutazone and most of the more recent anti-inflammatory analgesics are not only ulcerogenic, but also increase the risk of perforation in pre-existing peptic ulcers.

Complications of Diverticular Disease

61   Diverticulosis refers merely to the presence of diverticula, and is present in 30 per cent of the population over the age of 60, most of whom are symptomless. Diverticulitis, on the other hand, is the illness which develops when a segment of colon, usually the sigmoid, involved in diverticulosis, becomes the seat of an acute inflammatory process.

62   This is a nickname for acute diverticulitis. It refers to the similarity in the progression of symptoms and signs between these two conditions. Thus, in diverticulitis the patient often describes a vague lower abdominal pain which later localizes in the left iliac fossa, and on examination there is peritonism in the same area.

63   The diagnosis is usually fairly straightforward, with a story of localizing LIF pain, pyrexia, localized peritonism and perhaps, a tender mass. In females a tubo-ovarian infection should be excluded, and in both sexes evidence of perforation sought and the possibility of carcinoma remembered. Initially, treatment is conservative, comprising starvation, IV fluids, antibiotics (a cephalosporin, or gentamicin, with metronidazole) and analgesia. Usually the condition

settles over four to five days, although in a few, clinical signs and x-rays will suggest abscess formation or spreading peritonitis due to perforation, requiring urgent surgery. Following uneventful recovery from an uncomplicated episode a high fibre diet should be started and a barium enema, perhaps with colonoscopy, should be arranged to exclude a carcinoma. Repeated episodes of diverticulitis or failure to exclude carcinoma are indications for elective sigmoid colectomy.

64   The clinical picture presented by a pericolic abscess is similar to that of uncomplicated acute diverticulitis. The differences which suggest this diagnosis are the temperature, which begins to swing, and the presence of a tender mass, although this can occur without abscess formation. Later cases may develop overlying erythema. Clinical suspicion should be followed by ultrasonography. Once diagnosed, the abscess should be drained; this can usually be done by direct incision in the LIF, though sometimes formal laparotomy is needed to be sure of the diagnosis. Elective resection is usually performed at a later date.

65   Purulent and faecal. The former occurs when a pericolic abscess ruptures, while faecal peritonitis follows perforation of a diverticulum.

66   The stages are diagnosis, resuscitation and surgery which may itself be staged. The history of lower abdominal, and later generalized peritonitic pain, with physical signs of generalized peritonitis and, perhaps, shock, strongly suggest the diagnosis. Radiology will usually reveal free gas, often in large volumes. Resuscitation requires fluid replacement and broad spectrum antibiotics, with special care to recognize and deal with acute renal failure. In experienced hands, surgery usually involves peritoneal toilet followed by primary resection with either anastomosis and proximal loop colostomy, or Hartmann's procedure. For the less experienced, either the Paul-Mikulicz' operation or simply peritoneal toilet, local drainage and proximal colostomy will be performed, though the latter very conservative procedure is today much less used as the mortality due to leaving the diseased segment in situ is high. If the patient survives the acute episode, further surgery is normally required, either to close the stoma if primary resection was performed initially, or to resect the diseased segment and then close the stoma if simple drainage and colostomy had been the primary treatment.

67   Very poor. Untreated this is uniformly fatal, due to septicaemia and renal failure. Even after surgery,

especially if primary resection has not been possible, about 60 to 70 per cent of patients with faecal peritonitis will die. This is due to the usually advanced age and frequent intercurrent cardiorespiratory disease, coupled with the septic and renal complications of faecal peritonitis.

Acute pancreatitis

68 In this country about 60 per cent of cases occur in patients with gall-stones, and there is strong evidence for a causal relationship. A further 20 per cent are due to alcoholism, while the remainder are due to a myriad of factors, including steroid therapy, trauma (sometimes iatrogenic), hyperparathyroidism, mumps and several others. A few cases remain idiopathic. In countries where alcoholism is more prevalent, acute pancreatitis is correspondingly more common.

69 Although the presentation is rather variable, the usual picture is one of steadily increasing abdominal pain, peritonitic in nature, which may be epigastric or generalized. There is often a 'band-like' upper abdominal pain radiating to the back. The patient is usually nauseated and often vomits. On examination there is commonly a mild pyrexia, tachycardia and slight cyanosis. There is epigastric or generalized peritonism, sometimes to the extent of board-like rigidity. Bowel sounds may be diminished or absent.

70 Clinical suspicion will lead to taking of a blood sample to measure the serum amylase; if this is more than 1000 Somogyi units, the diagnosis is confirmed. If the serum amylase is less than 1000, pancreatitis is still possible, but other conditions such as perforated peptic ulcer and acute cholecystitis must be actively considered. Sometimes, with an amylase below 1000, and a high suspicion of perforated ulcer, laparotomy will be necessary, leading to macroscopic diagnosis of pancreatitis.

71 Initial management comprises the treatment of shock, and the recognition and treatment of any respiratory, renal and metabolic complications as early as possible. Treatment of shock entails fluid, protein and sometimes blood replacement, preferably with regular central venous pressure monitoring. Respiratory complications are frequent, and should be anticipated by blood gas analysis on admission and regularly thereafter. If the Po_2 falls below 70 mmHg, oxygen should be given. Further deterioration may require ventilation or tracheostomy. Renal failure, transient in the majority, occurs in up to 20 per cent. Bladder catheterization and hourly urine measurements are

mandatory from the outset. Oliguria should be actively treated by ensuring an adequate circulating volume followed by administration of diuretics. Other complications such as hypocalcaemia and clotting disorders must also be watched for. Pain relief is usually adequate with pethidine; peritoneal lavage is also useful in pain relief. Recently, some surgeons have advocated surgical drainage of the necrotic pancreas in the progressively deteriorating case. There is no proven place for the use of the antitryptic agent, Trasylol, or for glucagon.

72 The overall mortality is around 10 per cent. The mortality rate is higher in first than in recurrent attacks. It is also related to aetiology—traumatic and steroid-induced pancreatitis are particularly dangerous. Mortality increases with age.

Vascular conditions

73 Mesenteric embolism usually occurs in the superior mesenteric artery. The involved bowel, therefore, will be part or all of the mid-gut, the precise extent depending on how distally in the arterial system the embolus lodges. Thus, if it comes to rest in the trunk, all the bowel from the distal duodenum to the mid transverse colon will be at risk of infarction. Mesenteric infarction is an extremely serious condition, with a high mortality. 'Treatability' depends on the amount of bowel involved, and the age and general condition of the patient. If at laparotomy the bowel is dead from duodenum to splenic flexure it is probably best to close the abdomen. If, however, even 12 inches of small bowel is alive, then in the younger patient resection should be performed. However, subsequent nutrition may require permanent intravenous feeding, a formidable prospect, available in only a few units in this country.

74 Dead bowel is black, inert, has lost its serosal sheen, and remains motionless even when flicked with a finger. Severely ischaemic bowel may still be saved; its dark colour suggests that it is dead, but a few minutes wrapped in a hot pack will often lead to a return of contractility. If there is any doubt, ischaemic bowel is best assumed dead, and removed.

75 It is thought that this segment of bowel is usually affected because of the frequent lack of a marginal artery linking the superior and inferior mesenteric arteries at this point. Thus, any compromise of inferior mesenteric supply, either in the trunk or major branches, or in the smaller vessels around the bowel wall, will not be replaced by collateral supply from the superior mesenteric artery, leading to ischaemic changes in the bowel wall.

76 No. The diagnosis having been made on the basis of the age, frequently associated cardiovascular disease elsewhere, the history of sudden onset of bloody diarrhoea, localized left abdominal tenderness and diagnostic x-ray changes, the patient is treated conservatively with a good prospect of recovery within a few days. In a few the presentation is more dramatic, with evidence of peritonitis on admission, while in others this may develop after beginning conservative therapy. These patients require laparotomy and resection urgently. A few who recover on a conservative regimen later develop troublesome symptoms due to stricture—these also require surgery.

Gynaecological emergencies

77 Acute salpingitis, ruptured pyosalpinx, ovulatory bleeding, twisted ovarian cyst and ectopic pregnancy. Less commonly a twisted or degenerating fibroid, or a bleeding endometrioma can cause confusion.

78 The patient may be simply ill or in extremis, depending on whether the Fallopian tube has ruptured. If the bleeding is still contained in an intact tube, then the patient will typically give a history of one or two missed periods, with recent onset of hypogastric pain—usually colicky—and variable vaginal bleeding. On examination she will look uncomfortable, and there will be suprapubic tenderness, perhaps more on one side, and pelvic examination should reveal a tender forniceal mass. A much more dramatic, and potentially fatal, picture is seen after the tube has burst, releasing the tamponade, to allow free peritoneal haemorrhage. The patient will tell of a sudden onset of severe peritonitic pain, perhaps radiating to the shoulders. She will be pale, with a thready pulse. The abdomen may be distended and will be tender with guarding. Pelvic examination will be very uncomfortable, and the fornical mass should be palpable. This picture should lead to rapid diagnosis and life-saving surgery, preferably by a gynaecologist.

79 These two conditions may be difficult to distinguish; sometimes laparoscopy or even 'grid-iron' laparotomy is required in very doubtful cases. Distinction is usually possible, however, on clinical grounds. Salpingitis is not usually heralded by periumbilical pain, and salpingitic pain is normally suprapubic, often bilateral or even confined to the left side. A history of vaginal discharge should always be sought. On examination the site of tenderness in each disease corresponds to the site of pain; pelvic examination is

always necessary in young women, looking for vaginal discharge, cervical pain on manipulation and tender adnexae. A confident diagnosis of salpingitis will save the patient an operation.

Intestinal obstruction

80   In most cases, the cause will be found to be either an obstructed groin hernia or postoperative adhesions.

81   Intestinal obstruction disturbs the normal circulation of fluid between the blood and the bowel lumen. The eight litres of fluid secreted in the upper alimentary tract each day are normally mostly reabsorbed in the distal small bowel. In distal obstruction, not only does this absorption stop, but active secretion into the bowel occurs. Thus large volumes of fluid are sequestered in the bowel, leading to clinical dehydration even before vomiting begins.

82   It means literally what it says. It occurs in patients with intestinal obstruction—as the bowel progressively distends with fluid, it begins to empty itself into the stomach, leading to vomiting.

83   This is a particularly dangerous form of obstruction in which a loop of bowel is effectively obstructed at both ends, and is best exemplified by the obstructing annular colonic carcinoma. Normally the ileocaecal valve prevents reflex of colonic content into the ileum; in large bowel obstruction, ileocaecal continence prevents retrograde transmission of pressure into the small bowel. The closed loop of colon becomes grossly distended, and the high luminal pressure causes the occlusion of vessels in the bowel wall, leading to early perforation, usually in the caecum. Closed loop obstruction can be diagnosed on x-ray, and is an indication for urgent laparotomy. Luckily, the ileocaecal valve often fails to prevent reflux in large bowel obstruction, so that in such cases, the progression to caecal perforation is very unusual. Volvulus is another form of closed-loop obstruction.

84   This is essentially a clinical syndrome produced by incomplete intestinal obstruction. The patient complains of abdominal discomfort, perhaps with colic, and sometimes vomiting. The most important clinical feature is the continuance of bowel action, usually diarrhoea. On examination the abdomen may be modestly distended, and the bowel sounds obstructive. Radiology will show distended loops with fluid levels. Patients may present having been in this state for days, even a few weeks. Subacute obstruction is perhaps most commonly seen in slowly progressive conditions such as Crohn's disease, or peritoneal metastatic carcinoma, but it can occur in colorectal cancer or postoperative

adhesions. The place of surgery depends on the underlying pathology.

85 On admission, an estimate must be made of the abnormal fluid losses already suffered. This is is done by assessing the clinical state—vital signs, the state of the tongue, tissue elasticity—together with the length of history and frequency of vomiting. Clinical dehydration is not detectable until about two and a half litres have been lost in the average 70-kg man, while obvious dehydration will suggest a four and a half litre loss. The moribund patient may well be seven litres in deficit. As a rule of thumb, all the fluid can be assumed to have been equivalent to normal saline containing 20 mmol of potassium per litre. Fluid therapy in the first 24 hours will comprise the normal maintenance requirement, that is approximately three litres of fluid, including 140 mEq sodium and 40 mmol potassium, plus the estimated abnormal losses to date.

86 In one litre of normal saline there are 153 mmol each of sodium and chloride. In fact this solution, otherwise known as physiological saline, is not 'normal' in the chemical sense, nor quite isotonic.

87 This is a solution containing 131 mmol of sodium, 5 mmol of potassium, 4 mmol of calcium, 111 mmol of chloride and 29 mmol of lactate per litre. It was introduced as a mixture containing similar electrolyte concentrations to plasma.

88 There are two main features, the position of bowel loops and the mucosal pattern visible in the distended bowel. As a general rule, the large bowel will occupy the periphery of the abdomen though the transverse and sigmoid segments may lie centrally, especially when distended. Small bowel lies centrally, though it can appear to occupy the whole abdomen when distended. Mucosal pattern is a more useful pointer. Small bowel has a characteristic appearance—the mucosal folds, or valvulae conniventes, lie in regular sequence in the distended bowel, producing either multiple transverse bands or a series of ellipses. The haustra of the large bowel, on the other hand, appear as more widely spaced ingressions only partially crossing the lumen.

89 Knowing which parts of the bowel are distended helps decide the level of the obstruction and hence a plan for management. Distended small bowel alone, perhaps with a history of previous abdominal surgery and no evidence of external hernia, strongly suggests adhesion obstruction, which may be treated conservatively at first if the history is short, and there is no evidence of strangulation. Distended large bowel, indicating large bowel obstruction, strongly suggests

that surgery should be performed after adequate resuscitation, as all the most likely causes are best remedied by operation.

90 Full blood count, 'group and save', and urea and electrolytes. Although estimation of dehydration is mainly a clinical decision, the haemoglobin and blood urea help in this estimation. The electrolytes begin to change late in the natural history, so are a poor parameter of electrolyte depletion, but serve as a guide to progress on treatment. The white blood cell count is important when considering the possibility of strangulation. However, while a high white count is very worrying, a low count by no means excludes this complication.

91 Gallstone ileus. In this condition, gas enters the biliary tree via a cholecystenteric fistula—usually into the duodenum—caused by the erosion into the bowel of a large gall-stone. The stone then passes down the gut to impact, producing obstruction. Another possibility is that the cholecystenteric fistula is iatrogenic, performed to relieve obstructive jaundice. This should be ascertained from the history, especially if a scar is found. The obstruction may then simply be due to postoperative adhesions. However, one must not be distracted by the interesting x-ray from checking the hernial orifices.

92 Metabolic acidosis, developing as a result of dehydration and under-perfusion of body tissues, particularly the splanchnic circulation. Acidosis can be particularly severe in the presence of strangulated bowel. A precise assessment is made by arterial pH measurement and blood gas analysis. The mainstays of correction are adequate resuscitation and the removal of dead tissue. It is uncommon to need to give bicarbonate, but if the patient is shocked, or develops cardiac arrhythmias, an initial dose of 80 mmol of sodium bicarbonate is a sensible step.

93 The few useful signs all involve the presence of gas in abnormal positions. First, free gas in the peritoneal cavity indicates perforation, and strangulation or ischaemic perforation due to stretching of bowel wall are the likely causes. The other signs are more subtle; the presence of a thin line of gas a few millimetres lateral to the luminal gas shadow and parallel to its edge indicates gas in the bowel wall, and is a sure sign of dead bowel. Finally, retroperitoneal gas, or bubbles around the bulge of a groin hernia, also indicate dead bowel. All these signs are urgent indications for operation.

94 Plain abdominal films are important in diagnosis, but barium enema offers definitive diagnosis and, in some

cases, a mode of treatment. The plain films will confirm intestinal obstruction and also the characteristic absence of gas in the right abdomen. Barium enema will demonstrate an ileocolic intussusception—the classical 'coil-spring' appearance produced as the barium spreads between the advancing intussusception and the bowel wall, is usually seen. So long as the history is no longer than 24 hours, and there is no clinical suspicion of gangrene, the hydrostatic pressure transmitted by barium enema can be used to reduce an intussusception.

95 Any gynaecological procedure, or appendicectomy.

96 As a general rule, acute intestinal obstruction is an indication for surgery after initial resuscitation. However, adhesion obstruction, especially if recurrent, is best treated conservatively at first, unless there is a long history or any worry at all about strangulation. The advantages of conservatism are that many cases will settle on nasogastric suction and IV fluids, and that further surgery, while relieving the obstruction, may well make the adhesions worse, inviting future problems. If a conservative approach is used a very careful watch for deterioration is imperative, and anyway, if no improvement is seen within, say 36 hours, then surgery is necessary.

97 No. Although usually a sign of intestinal obstruction, in very thin people, especially if old or emaciated, the abdominal wall can be so thin that normal peristalsis may be visible.

98 Yes—'bolus' and 'Stammer's loop' obstructions. Bolus obstruction, due to the impaction of a mass of undigested food in the distal small bowel, is especially liable after gastrectomy as access to the small bowel is so rapid. Avoidance of pithy fruit and careful mastication should be impressed upon gastrectomy patients. Stammer's loop obstruction occurs when a variable length of small bowel becomes twisted around the afferent and efferent loops of the antecolic gastrojejunal anastomosis. This usually occurs within three weeks of gastrectomy, and presents with the features of high small bowel obstruction. Early surgery is mandatory once the diagnosis is made.

99 Yes, there is a procedure called Noble's plication, in which the small bowel is carefully mobilized and then sutured in a 'step ladder' or 'jumping cracker' configuration, so that it lies in the abdomen in a fixed, hopefully trouble-free, position.

100 Certain clinical pointers do exist, but none is completely reliable. Strangulation sometimes produces a peritonitic, constant pain superimposed on the colic.

On examination the development of tenderness, especially if a mass is palpable, is a worrying sign, as are pyrexia and tachycardia over 100 per minute. Hypotension, especially with pyrexia, is more common if strangulation has occurred.

101 The site of pain and the timing of onset of vomiting and absolute constipation differ. Small bowel obstruction usually causes colicky pain in the epigastrium or periumbilical area, while large bowel colic is likely to be hypogastric. Vomiting begins soon after the onset of pain in high small bowel obstruction, but for progressively more distal obstruction the vomiting occurs later, so that in distal large bowel obstruction this symptom may not appear at all. Constipation on the other hand has the opposite relationship—it is noticed almost immediately in sigmoid obstruction, while normal bowel activity may continue for 24 hours in high small bowel obstruction.

102 Carcinoma.

103 Spurious means inappropriate or misleading. Spurious diarrhoea is a symptom of incipient large bowel obstruction. The classical story in spurious diarrhoea is one of a recurring cycle of several days of constipation, followed by an episode of loose, even incontinent bowel actions. The diarrhoea occurs because the only motion able to creep past the obstruction is liquid stool. It is important to differentiate this pattern of bowel habit from infective diarrhoea and colitis, in which diarrhoea is usually continual.

104 Yes, several. First, as the most common cause of large bowel obstruction is carcinoma, it is extremely unlikely that the obstruction will settle spontaneously. Therefore, a prolonged period of non-operative treatment is liable to lead to fluid balance problems, and the various complications related to bed rest, such as DVT. Another important possibility is the development of closed loop obstruction, with the risk of perforation. Therefore, in a case of large bowel obstruction, once adequate resuscitation has been performed, it is best to proceed to surgery without undue delay.

105 This is a form of large bowel obstruction, due to twisting of the sigmoid colon around the axis of its mesocolon. The sigmoid colon thus forms a closed loop, and may become massively distended, filling the abdomen. At presentation the patient may give a history of similar previous episodes, which may have settled spontaneously. This condition seems to be more common amongst patients in mental institutions.

106 After adequate resuscitation, the patient requires an operation, the prime aim of which is to relieve the obstruction. In inexperienced hands, the emergency operation should be a laparotomy to confirm the diagnosis and to fashion a defunctioning transverse colostomy. Definitive resection and colostomy closure follow as one or two stages in the ensuing weeks. For more experienced surgeons the emergency procedure will usually involve the resection of the carcinoma. There is an increased risk of anastomotic breakdown in this setting as the bowel is distended and usually loaded with faeces, so the surgeon will usually fashion a proximal temporary colostomy to protect the anastomosis.

107 This is a condition in which the patient appears to be suffering from mechanical obstruction, while in fact no obstruction is present. The patient often has the classical symptoms, and examination may reveal distension and obstructed bowel sounds. X-rays will show distended small and/or large bowel. The tell-tale signs of the true diagnosis, are the findings of a ballooned rectum on digital examination and gas extending down to the rectum on x-ray. Patients with this condition are often found to be on drugs which can affect bowel motility, such as anti-Parkinsonian medication. These cases usually settle on conservative management, though most surgeons will 'accidentally' open a patient before making the diagnosis at some time in their career.

108 This is the term applied by surgeons to a very small primary colonic tumour sometimes found at laparotomy for obstruction. The lesion is so small that at first sight the obstruction looks as though it could simply be due to ligature—or string—tied tightly around the colon.

Abdominal trauma

109 This physical sign indicates that the abdominal contents have been compressed between the vehicle tyre and the vertebral column, and is an absolute indication for laparotomy; it is highly likely that a major injury to an abdominal viscus will be found, especially the bowel, mesentery or pancreas.

110 This clinical picture strongly suggests traumatic haemobilia. In this condition, trauma to the liver, blunt or sharp, causes intrahepatic haemorrhage leading to local necrosis and sepsis, which may be enough to induce jaundice. Material from the necrotic haematoma then bursts into the biliary tree, perhaps at the site of a knife injury to a duct, and hence into the bowel. Further haemorrhage from the injured area then leads to the passage of malaena.

111 In most patients there will be a history of blunt abdominal or lower chest trauma within the previous few hours, though in some it may have occurred several days previously. They will complain of variably severe abdominal pain, worse on movement, and often referred to the left shoulder. On examination there will be pallor and signs of hypovolaemia. Abdominal examination will reveal local or generalized tenderness and diminished bowel sounds.

112 As the nerves supplying the abdominal wall are usually T8 to T12, trauma to the chest wall can bruise or damage these nerves as they pass along the line of the ribs. This can produce reflex spasm of the abdominal wall musculature, mimicking the picture produced by intra-abdominal injury, even when all is well within the peritoneum.

113 Any penetrating wound up to the level of the sixth rib, or roughly the level of the nipples, may have entered the abdomen, as the domes of the diaphragm reach up to this level.

114 The organs most likely to be injured by a seat belt are those that are relatively fixed in position within the abdomen, so that they cannot slip out of the way when squeezed by the belt, and especially those lying in front of the spinal column. Thus the organs most at risk are the stomach and bladder (especially when either is full) the duodenum, pancreas and small bowel with its mesentery.

115 While stab wounds to the abdomen cause visceral injury in only 30 per cent of cases, bullet wounds from a hand gun almost always produce some visceral damage, while velocity missiles always produce major destruction along the bullet track. A knife blade often deflects movable viscera as it enters the abdomen, though relatively fixed structures are more vulnerable; low-velocity bullets, as from a hand gun, dissipate their kinetic energy rapidly as they penetrate, and may be deflected by important structures. High-velocity bullets, however, have enormous energy, causing explosive destruction of tissue several centimetres each side of the track, often causing fatal injury.

116 A stab wound involving the anterior wall of the stomach may well have penetrated the posterior wall also, perhaps even injuring the pancreas. Therefore these structures must always be inspected by formal opening of the lesser sac—otherwise these life-threatening injuries may be missed.

117 This is a collection of blood enclosed within the capsule of the spleen, developing as a result of blunt trauma. Its significance is that, although the patient may have

minimal symptoms and signs of splenic injury, the haematoma can rupture several days after the initial trauma, accompanied by further haemorrhage from the damaged parenchyma, and this can be serious or even fatal. If such an injury is suspected the patient should be observed in hospital, and subjected to radio-isotope scanning of the spleen, which may demonstrate the haematoma as a 'cold' defect in the splenic image.

118 Severe blunt trauma to the abdomen can cause a rupture of the diaphragm due to the sudden rise in intra-abdominal pressure—abdominal organs may then pass into the chest, causing a major impairment to vital capacity and ventilatory efficiency. The left diaphragm is damaged more often than the right, which is protected by the liver; stomach, colon and small bowel can all pass up into the chest.

119 Peritoneal lavage is the most sensitive and reliable way of confirming intraperitoneal haemorrhage. A peritoneal dialysis cannula is inserted through the linea alba below the umbilicus after making sure the bladder is empty. Blood may issue directly from the cannula, in which case the haemorrhage is proven. More often, it is necessary to run in 500 ml of saline, and then to syphon it out again by putting the infusion bag onto the floor while still connected. Blood staining of the fluid is a reliable indicator of a bleed.

120 There are no pathognomonic radiological signs of ruptured spleen, but useful pointers are: posterior fractures of the left lower ribs, which lie behind the spleen; rightward shift of the gastric air bubble; fluid between coils of intestine; and elevation of the left diaphragm.

121 This test is unreliable and hence can lead to bad decisions. Moreover, it is evidence of visceral damage rather than merely of peritoneal penetration which is important, so probing of the wound need never be considered.

122 Chest x-ray will show loss of the normally clear line of the diaphragm, usually on the left, with partial collapse of the lung and perhaps a fluid level within a displaced abdominal viscus. Free gas, due to pneumothorax or ruptured viscus, may also be seen.

123 Bullet wounds to the abdomen always require laparotomy due to the high likelihood of visceral damage. Blunt trauma and stab wounds require exploration only when careful initial or subsequent clinical and radiological examination provide any evidence suggesting visceral injury.

124 This group of patients will include those with blunt trauma or stab wounds in whom there is no evidence of visceral damage on admission. They require careful monitoring, watching for evidence of intraperitoneal haemorrhage or leakage from a hollow viscus. Having taken blood for cross-matching and base line investigations, the vital signs are monitored hourly to begin with, and the abdomen examined frequently for signs of peritoneal irritation. Any change suggesting visceral damage should lead to operation. If all is stable at 48 hours the patient can usually be discharged, but if there is a possibility of intrahepatic or intrasplenic injury, a longer watch should be kept, and ultrasound or isotope scanning performed.

125 The safest surgical manoeuvre in this situation is exteriorization of the injured segment to form a temporary colostomy, as primary repair of a wound in a bowel loaded with faeces is liable to break down, causing peritonitis. If the bowel injury is ragged, a resection will be performed, either with anastomosis and proximal colostomy or with temporary exteriorization of the two ends.

126 Ampicillin, tobramycin and metronidazole; this combination will cover the broad spectrum of organisms likely to be spilt from a lacerated large bowel. Some surgeons might replace ampicillin and tobramycin with a cephalosporin such as cefoxitin or cephradine.

127 The surgeon will first try to decide whether the external appearance of the liver reflects the internal damage—sometimes a small surface laceration hides an extensive intrahepatic haematoma with major vessel damage and major devitalization of liver tissue. If bleeding is occurring, he may try to control it temporarily, while he assesses the injury, by placing a non-crushing clamp on the structures in the free edge of the lesser omentum—Pringle's manoeuvre. If the injury is considered local, bleeding is controlled and the liver wound may be closed with sutures or omentum. If the internal damage is more major, then either a wedge resection to remove dead and bruised tissue or even a right hepatic lobectomy will be performed.

General surgical care

Water, electrolytes and nutrition

128 About 1200 ml of water is taken in by drinking. The water content of solid food contributes about a litre and a further 300 ml on average is generated in the course of

metabolism. The normal urine output is of the order of 1500 ml with about 900 ml insensible loss from breathing and perspiration in a temperate climate, and about 100 ml lost in faeces.

129   Water is required to match the predicted losses, to correct a pre-existing deficit and to correct any additional losses during the 24 hours. The predicted losses should allow 1500 ml for urine and 1000 ml for insensible loss. Since the operation was routine it is likely that the patient left the operating theatre in balance but it is likely that there will be some addition to be made for nasogastric aspirate or other drainage. A total allowance of 3 litres is fairly typical.

130   There may be clinical evidence of water deficit or excess at the outset and a correction for this should be made in the fluid orders for the next period. All abnormal losses from fistulae, drains, diarrhoea and nasogastric aspiration must be accounted for and the fluid charts from the previous 24 hours should contain this information. Increased insensible loss due to fever or tachypnoea should be allowed for. The urine output should be measured and if it is low the possibility of renal failure must be carefully considered before ordering extra fluid.

131   A typical intake of sodium is 75 to 100 mmol but it is highly variable from day to day and from one individual to another. The healthy kidney can conserve or excrete sodium over a very wide range by producing urine containing few millimoles or several hundred millimoles of sodium per day.

132   This is below the normal range which is about 135 to 145 mmol. This is rarely due to true sodium depletion but more commonly to an excess of circulating water, either infused as 5 per cent dextrose, or the result of innappropriate ADH secretion. Apparent hyponatraemia can occur if there is an unusually large proportion of non-aqueous material in the serum sample, such as fat or protein.

133   A high serum sodium may be due to excessive infusion of sodium chloride, when there is usually oedema due to water retention. Alternatively, it can occur with water depletion; the hypernatraemia is unlikely to be gross except in diabetes insipidus, for instance with a basal skull fracture.

134   About 80 mmol of potassium per day is lost in the urine which accounts for virtually all the daily loss. The minimum urinary potassium loss is about 20 mmol/litre.

135 Abnormal losses from the gastro-intestinal tract over a long period can result in hypokalaemia. Examples are prolonged nasogastric aspiration, loss from fistulae, and diarrhoea in particular due to ulcerative colitis or villous tumours. Prolonged treatment with some diuretics can cause potassium depletion. Treatment of diabetic coma with insulin results in intracellular movement of potassium causing an acutely low serum potassium. Cardiac dysrhythmias, including ventricular fibrillation, may result. Lesser but more common consequences are general lethargy and muscular weakness.

136 A potassium of this level is dangerous because it may result in asystolic arrest, so it should be brought down. The quickest way to do this is by injecting a mixture of 25 g glucose and 10 units of insulin. This is only a temporary measure and if the underlying cause is renal failure peritoneal dialysis should be instituted.

137 The aspirate is a mixture of gastric, pancreatic and small bowel secretions and bile and is likely to contain 100 to 150 mmol/litre of sodium and 5 to 10 mmol/litre of potassium. A replacement regimen of volume for volume normal saline with 10 mmol of potassium chloride added to each litre should be given in addition to other fluids. This should be modified in the light of clinical progress and the results of serum electrolyte estimations. Electrolytes can also be measured in aliquots of the aspirate to confirm the initial estimates.

138 As a rule of thumb replacement with normal saline with 10 mmol per litre of potassium chloride should be instigated. This should be added to the daily ration allowed for urinary and insensible loss. However, as this may require chronic management a day by day balance should be calculated, and the patient's clinical state assessed to ensure that the overall water balance is being maintained. Similarly measurements of electrolytes in the urine and in aliquots of the fistula fluid can be used to produce a balance sheet for the electrolytes. Measurement of serum electrolytes may only identify gross discrepancies because of the ability of the kidneys to correct for inappropriate fluid loss.

139 The main danger in infusing potassium chloride is that it is easy to produce a transient hyperkalaemia which may cause cardiac arrest. The best way to prevent this is to avoid high concentrations of potassium and not to infuse more than 20 mmol per hour. Potassium can also produce ischaemic

ulceration of the skin if allowed to run into the tissues.

140 About half the serum calcium is protein bound, about 45 per cent is ionized and the remainder is present in solution but complexed with organic ions such as citrate.

141 Calcium is mobilized from bones in hyperparathyroidism and in malignant disease such as myelomatosis or advanced breast carcinoma. There may be increased absorption in vitamin D overdosage, sarcoid or milk alkali syndrome. Severe hypercalcaemia results in coma and anuria. Less severe, chronic hypercalcaemia causes calcification in the kidneys, constipation, vomiting and a generalized feeling of illness and depression.

142 Vomiting over a long period or nasogastric aspiration when the fluid is replaced with magnesium-free solutions can result in magnesium depletion. The loop diuretics can also have this effect.

143 Following surgery there is an expected catabolic period when the body's protein is used to provide energy. A patient who is already cachectic tolerates this poorly and may become acidotic with a rising urea. Healing and resistance to infection may be poor.

144 For the average adult an IV regime should contain 2000 to 3000 calories, a balanced supply of the essential amino acids to give 10 to 20 g of nitrogen, the essential fatty acids, vitamins and trace elements in addition to the usual ration of water and electrolytes. The calories can be supplied as glucose alone, adding insulin if required, or mixtures of ethanol, sorbitol and fat suspensions can also be used.

145 Infection on the intravenous feeding catheter occurs readily unless great care is taken. The patient can be made hyperosmolar, hyperglycaemic or forced into lactic acidosis depending on which solution is used and how fast it is given.

Management of the circulation

146 Shock is a term used to indicate failure of the circulatory system. The typical features are pallor, cold peripheries, sweating, tachycardia, oliguria and hypotension. The causes include loss of circulating volume due to acute haemorrhage; acute depletion of extracellular fluid due to conditions such as intestinal obstruction or burns; acute severe heart failure, when it is called cardiogenic shock; or sudden changes in the peripheral resistance or permeability as occurs in Gram-negative septicaemia.

147 The term hypovolaemia means that there is insufficient fluid in the vascular compartment to maintain an adequate circulation. In addition to evidence of poor circulation as witnessed by tachycardia, cool peripheries, small volume peripheral pulses, reduced urine output and eventually arterial hypotension there should also be evidence of reduced filling pressures to make the diagnosis—a low jugular venous pressure or, more reliably, a low central venous pressure indicates that there is hypovolaemic rather than cardiogenic shock. The volume mismatch is usually due to loss of intravascular volume but occasionally it is due to inappropriate dilatation of the vessels.

148 Blood, plasma protein fraction, dextran, gelatin (Haemaccel), electrolyte and glucose solutions can all be used to expand the circulation. Electrolyte and glucose solutions are readily available and are, in relatively small volumes, fairly innocuous but they do not stay in the circulation and can produce salt or water overload if used to maintain circulating volume. The larger molecular weight solutions stay in the circulation longer but do not carry oxygen, and dextran may cause bleeding abnormalities. Blood loss if more than a litre is best replaced with blood. This may not be immediately available, needs cross-matching and may cause reactions.

149 The central venous pressure is a measure of the right atrial pressure and therefore of the filling pressure of the heart. It indicates the volume in the circulation, and it indicates when to continue and when to stop transfusion in a volume depleted patient. If, in spite of a central venous pressure of 10 to 15 cm, the circulation is still inadequate, there is an additional, probably cardiac cause.

150 An intravenous catheter must be introduced into the right atrium or a central vein close to it. The most commonly used routes are internal jugular and subclavian veins, and relatively short catheters about 15 cm long can be introduced percutaneously in the neck or below the clavicle. Alternatively, longer lines can be threaded up from the arm. The catheter is connected to a giving set with a three-way tap in the system so that the patient's venous circulation can form one side of a U-tube manometer and the pressure read off directly in centimetres of water using the estimated position of the right atrium in the mid chest as zero.

151 Oliguria means a reduced amount of urine. A urine output of 500 ml or less in 24 hours should cause

concern. If the patient is catheterized and the urine output is being monitored more closely, an output of under 0.5 ml/kg/hr for two or more consecutive hours calls for action.

152 The first step is to make sure that the flow and pressure to the kidney are satisfactory, so the circulatory system should be assessed. Once this has been done the urine output can be stimulated if necessary using a diuretic or osmotic agent such as mannitol beginning with a low dose. This is particularly appropriate if there is a recognized factor such as jaundice or haemolysis when maintaining urine flow may be important.

153 Inadequate renal perfusion, septicaemia, jaundice, certain antibiotics including cephalosporins and aminoglycosides, haemoglobin from mismatched transfusions and myoglobin from crush injuries are factors that may contribute to the development of acute renal failure.

154 As soon as it is established that there is renal failure on the grounds that the urine output remains minimal or absent in spite of adequate perfusion, and a trial of diuretics has failed to produce a response, the fluid intake should be restricted. Only enough should be given to cover the insensible loss and other non-renal losses. A diet low in protein but with sufficient calories to minimize catabolism is given. The bladder catheter should be removed to reduce the risk of infection. Dialysis may be required and should be instituted to treat dangerously high potassium, acidosis, fluid overload or a progressively rising urea. The diuretic phase may follow after a few days or two to three weeks, when adequate fluid replacement becomes the major problem.

155 Postoperative hypertension is hazardous because it increases the risks of bleeding at the operation site, can precipitate intracerebral bleeding and puts an increased work load on the left ventricle. The commonest cause is pain which should be assessed and relieved. Carbon dioxide retention due to respiratory difficulty should be dealt with if present. If severe hypertension persists, for example a diastolic pressure sustained at 120 mmHg, it should be treated with vasodilator drugs such as a nitroprusside infusion and ideally this should be undertaken with the support of an intensive care unit.

156 Blood transfusion can cause circulatory problems, transfusion reactions or infection. The infusion of any solution which expands the blood volume can overload

the circulation and cause heart failure and pulmonary oedema. If there is mismatch the reaction may include pyrexia, rash and hypotension. Haemolysis which releases haemoglobin into the circulation may result in acute renal failure if not promptly treated. Transfused blood can also be the source of infection, most notably with serum hepatitis, although this is now carefully screened.

157 Blood should be taken for the standard clotting tests and for a platelet count and the results discussed with the haematologist. The problem may be in the clotting factors, platelets, due to defibrination, or in the vessels themselves. The commonest cause is depletion of clotting factors and platelets due to replacement of surgical blood loss with old stored blood. This is treated with fresh frozen plasma, platelet concentrates or fresh blood. The prothrombin time is abnormal with liver disease and oral anticoagulants. The kaolin-cephalin time is abnormal in haemophilia. Clotting factor deficiencies of this kind can be corrected with a fresh frozen plasma from the transfusion laboratory. A platelet count below 20 000 per mm^3 can be responsible for a prolonged bleeding time but even if the count is normal, the activity may be reduced, as occurs with aspirin, and platelet concentrates may be necessary.

Postoperative complications

158 Infection is the most likely explanation and the wound, the chest and the bladder are possible sites. Deep infection related to the operation site must be considered. Another possibility is deep vein thrombosis, even in the absence of physical signs.

159 Bacteriological specimens should be obtained from the sputum and urine. Wound, faeces and blood cultures may also be indicated. A chest x-ray should be taken. A white cell count and differential should be done. Any clinical leads should be followed, such as ankle oedema or calf tenderness, and appropriate special investigations arranged.

160 A swinging pyrexia suggests that there are episodes of bacteraemia and the most likely source is an abscess. The wound, pelvis or under the diaphragm are the most likely sites.

161 Haematoma, bacterial contamination, ischaemia, necrosis, and foreign material contribute to wound infection. These all provide a culture medium which is kept around 37°C encouraging bacterial growth.

162 The anaerobic organisms play a large part in about 80 per cent of infections complicating large bowel surgery and are not identified unless specific techniques are employed.

163 The first job is to drain the abscess. In most instances this is done surgically and a drain is left in the cavity to ensure that it does not reaccumulate. Inaccessible abscesses can be treated these days by aspiration through a wide bore needle but the general rules still apply. Antibiotics are a valuable adjunct to deal with associated bacteraemia and cellulitis but are not a routine part of the treatment of an abscess.

164 Sputum retention, patchy atelectasis and lobar consolidation may occur after major surgery. The secretions are thick after anaesthesia and pain reduces depth of ventilation and inhibits coughing; these contribute to the pulmonary complications. The areas of atelectasis permit arteriovenous shunting and result in hypoxia.

165 The patient should be made as fit as possible pre-operatively by intensive physiotherapy and, if possible, surgery should be avoided in the winter months. Postoperative analgesic measures, local and systemic, help to preserve coughing but over-sedation must be avoided. Humidification helps to clear sputum.

166 Areas of lung which are not ventilated but still receive pulmonary blood flow represent areas of right to left shunt and cause arterial hypoxia. This can be recognized by the association of low Po_2 with a relatively low Pco_2 which happens because the hypoxia stimulates respiration and carbon dioxide is blown off to below normal levels.

167 Although chest infection can cause haemoptysis, pulmonary infarction due to thrombo-embolism is the probable diagnosis. If on the basis of the overall clinical picture this looks likely, urgent lower limb phlebography should be performed to confirm deep vein thrombosis so that treatment aimed at preventing further embolism may be started. The patient should then be heparinized, anticoagulation with Warfarin initiated, and local measures such as use of elasticated stockings used to discourage further thrombus formation. More detailed investigations to confirm pulmonary embolism such as ventilation/perfusion scans may follow but will not alter management in this particular clinical situation.

168 Virchow's triad comprises changes in vessel walls, changes in blood flow and changes in the composition of the blood; these three cause deep vein thrombosis.

They are represented in the patient as local pressure on the calf vessels or pelvic vessels during surgery; venous stasis due to immobility; and increased number and adhesiveness of platelets.

169   While many are asymptomatic, the first clue may be a pulmonary embolus. The leg oedema, particularly unilateral, calf pain, tenderness, and an unexplained low grade fever may all suggest deep vein thrombosis. The diagnosis is confirmed definitively by phlebography.

170   The clinical features depend on whether the embolism is massive, presenting with gross circulatory abnormalities, or smaller, presenting as pulmonary infarction. Massive pulmonary embolism causes sudden severe breathlessness associated with cyanosis, tachycardia, poor peripheral circulation and raised jugular venous pressure. All these features are due to sudden severe obstruction to blood flow in the pulmonary artery. Smaller emboli present as one or more episodes of haemoptysis and pleuritic pain associated with a rub. In addition there may be signs of right ventricular obstruction in addition.

171   The diagnosis is confirmed by pulmonary angiography or ventilation/perfusion lung scans. A pulmonary angiogram is required if surgery is considered essential in massive pulmonary embolism and will confirm the diagnosis and demonstrate the position and extent of the thrombus. The demonstration of areas of unperfused lung that are otherwise normal on the chest x-ray confirms and shows the distribution of smaller, possibly multiple, and less immediately life-threatening emboli.

172   Urgent heparinization is the treatment of choice in pulmonary embolism. In a small minority of patients who survive massive emboli but remain in a critical circulatory state, surgical removal, preferably on bypass, may be successful. Streptokinase infusion, particularly directly into the pulmonary artery, can succeed but is associated with troublesome complications.

173   Perioperative thrombus formation in the legs must be prevented. Subcutaneous heparin given with the premedication and twice daily in the postoperative period has been proven to reduce the risk. Local measures such as 'anti-embolism' stockings reduce venous stasis. The patient is kept mobile before and as soon as possible after surgery. Local calf pressure is avoided on the operating table and during the convalescence. Dehydration is avoided.

174 If there is evidence of poor peripheral circulation, poor urine output or arterial hypotension in spite of adequate filling pressures as judged from the jugular venous pulse or a CVP line, a myocardial cause should be suspected. A 12-lead ECG and a series of cardiac enzymes over the next three days will confirm the diagnosis of myocardial infarction.

175 Severe pain is a cause of tachycardia. If this has been excluded the major causes are volume deficit and cardiopulmonary problems. The differential diagnosis depends basically on two things: what is the rhythm and what is the venous pressure? If the patient is in sinus rhythm and the venous pressure is low the circulation is underfilled. This should be rapidly corrected and any underlying cause such as haemorrhage dealt with. If there is a new abnormality in the rhythm such as atrial fibrillation, which may be precipitated by surgery, this should be treated appropriately. If there is sinus tachycardia with a high CVP this suggests a myocardial problem.

176 The circulation must be maintained and the blood oxygenated with the absolute minimum of delay if there is to be any chance of success. The sequence of priorities is important. Look at the patient quickly checking for carotid pulse or heart sounds and for any obvious, reversible cause such as an obstructed airway. A call for help is issued as soon as a genuine emergency is confirmed, which should take only a second or two, and cardiac massage started with adequate force and rate. After four or five seconds give the first couple of breaths of mouth-to-mouth respiration. Maintain massage and ventilation as long as you are on your own. As help arrives delegate and share tasks according to the relative experience of the personnel available. Record the sequence of events as accurately as possible after the crisis is over if you were first on the scene.

177 The blood loss must be replaced and the bleeding stopped. If cross-matched blood is available this should be given at a rate appropriate for the circulatory state and the rate of loss. Otherwise, the next most suitable fluid available should be given. A member of the surgical team should make an urgent decision about re-exploration of the operation site, recognizing that the patient will stand further anaesthesia and surgery better if some time can be spent on resuscitation.

'Lumps and bumps'

178 On inspection the size, shape, smoothness or irregularity of its outline and its position in relation to anatomical landmarks may be noted. On palpation these findings can be confirmed and whether the lump is hard or soft, uniform or lobulated, hot or cold can be established. Its relationship to superficial and deep anatomical structures can be tested and the extent of tethering to these layers and the tests for fluctuance and transillumination performed.

179 To elicit fluctuance the lump is secured across a diameter between two fingers of one hand and gently pressed with the fingers of the other hand. Transmitted pressure to the securing fingers is interpreted as fluctuance.

180 Tethering to the overlying skin or to deeper tissues may indicate invasion and therefore malignancy.

181 This is a useful trick to determine what layer a lump is in. If the muscles are tensed a superficial lump is more easily palpable while the borders of a deep lump become obscured.

182 A lump filled with clear fluid which is not too deeply situated will transmit light.

183 The lump would be red, hot, tense and tender.

184 A deep abscess should be suspected in a patient with spikes of fever, sometimes preceded by rigors and recurring every few hours. If it is sufficiently superficial a red, hot, tense and tender lump will usually be apparent. Abscesses require drainage.

185 Cellulitis is a spreading infection which tracks along subcutaneously or follows fascial planes. It is due to *Streptococcus* which produces an enzyme called streptokinase which breaks down fibrin and prevents localization of the infection.

186 A boil is an infection originating in a hair follicle. There is a single abscess cavity just deep to the skin with surrounding inflammation. It discharges spontaneously through a central area of skin softening and then typically resolves quite promptly. A carbuncle is an area of infection in the subcutaneous tissues. There is more generalized necrosis and the pus is usually loculated in several smaller abscess cavities. The overlying skin may be lost as a slough leaving a necrotic area.

187 This description fits a lipoma, a lobulated, thinly encapsulated mass of fat which most commonly occurs superficially but can occur almost anywhere in the body. It is a benign lesion.

188 In Dercum's disease there are multiple, tender lipomata which are found particularly on the trunk.

189 A sebaceous cyst is found most commonly on the scalp. It appears hemispherical with smooth borders and a central punctum. It moves with the skin but is not fixed deeply. It is fluctuant but does not transilluminate.

190 Nobody knows. It is therefore difficult to evaluate the effectiveness of new treatments. They are due to a virus and it seems likely that variations in the body's immunological state may be responsible for the sometimes sudden and dramatic clearance of a crop of warts.

191 Keloid is overgrowth of skin in a scar. Scar hypertrophy is common but resolves within a few months, whereas true keloid progresses for a year or more and never fully resolves. It is more common in black skin.

192 'T' stands for tumour, 'N' for nodes and 'M' for metastases. T–0 indicates an undetected primary, while T-3 indicates a large or locally advanced primary. N–0 to N–3 indicate from no nodal involvement through anatomically more extensive lymphatic spread. M–0 means no detected distant metastases and M–1 means that metastases have been located. The disease is classified under these headings to permit standardization of treatment and comparison between groups.

193 Increase in size, ulceration, deepening colour, itching, bleeding or a halo of pigmentation are all reasons to suspect malignant melanoma in a pre-existing mole.

194 The diagnosis is confirmed histologically and this should be done by excision biopsy with at least a centimetre margin. The surgeon is prepared to proceed to a much wider clearance as soon as the diagnosis is known.

195 Age, sunshine, irradiation and exposure of the skin to chemical irritants such as dyes, tar and soot can all predipose to the development of skin cancer. It can also develop in areas of senile keratosis or in an ulcer when it is known as Marjolin's ulcer.

196 The ulcer has rolled edges with a pearly appearance and the centre scabs over and breaks down from time

to time. They are nearly always on the face, above the level of the mouth and quite commonly near the eye or nose. Local erosion (as a rat might gnaw) is a feature, which is why the name 'rodent ulcer' was given to this lesion, histologically a basal cell carcinoma.

197 The enlargement can be due to malignant disease, either primary or secondary, or to infection which may be regional or generalized. Primary malignant conditions of lymph nodes include Hodgkin's disease and other lymphomas, although the axilla is one of the less common sites. Breast carcinoma is the commonest cause of secondary malignancy in the axilla. Infections involving the hand or arm may spread via the lymphatics and present with axillary lymphadenitis—cat scratch fever is in this group. Any of the conditions causing generalized lymphadenitis, such as glandular fever, should be included in the differential diagnosis although other node groups are usually involved.

198 A pharyngeal pouch can give this history, as can a stone in the submandibular duct. The distinction can be made with a carefully taken history. The salivary gland swelling is due to salivation alone and it resolves spontaneously whereas a pouch fills with food during a meal and the swelling persists until this is regurgitated or emptied in some way.

199 The differential diagnosis includes primary or secondary malignancy and infection, which is likely to be in the area of the lymphatic drainage. Hodgkin's disease and the lymphomas often present this way. Primary carcinoma of the larynx, nasopharynx, tongue and thyroid are among the causes of secondary malignancy. Any infection in the drainage area can cause this; tuberculosis should not be forgotten.

200 The commonest causes of a tender lump in the groin are strangulated hernia and inflamed lymph nodes. A femoral hernia should always be considered and, of the groin herniae, is the most likely to present in this way. Lymphadenitis or abscess formation may follow infection somewhere in the limb. Less common causes include malignancy, an ectopic testis and femoral artery aneurysm.

201 This was the first human tumour in which there appeared to be a transmissible causative agent. The tumour is only found in areas which share a particular climate and have in common the malaria mosquito which might act as a vector.

202 Torsion of the testis and acute epididymo-orchitis are two conditions that present in this way. The differential diagnosis is usually difficult so the rule is that all tender scrotal swellings should be seen by a surgeon with a view to immediate surgical exploration. However, over the age of about 25 torsion does not occur, so exploration is not necessary in this age group. A less common condition is torsion of the hydatid of Morgagni.

Hernia

203 The pubic tubercle and the pubic crest medial to it are the surface landmarks of the superficial inguinal ring. The lateral crus is attached to the pubic tubercle which is palpated by invaginating the scrotum behind the cord. The triangular shaped 'ring' lies immediately above and medial to it with the pubic crest forming its inferior border.

204 The deep ring is bounded laterally and inferiorly by transversus muscle and its attachment to the inguinal ligament. Above and medially is the transversalis fascia. Medially the fascia is condensed over the inferior epigastric vessels which are an important surgical landmark.

205 The spermatic cord includes the vas deferens with its artery and lymphatics, the testicular artery, accompanying sympathetic fibres and the pampiniform plexus of veins. The cord has three coverings: the internal spermatic fascia derived from the transversalis fascia; the cremasteric fascia from the external oblique; and the external spermatic fascia from the external oblique aponeurosis. The cord is not really complete until it leaves the superficial ring.

206 Anteriorly is the inguinal ligament, posteriorly the thickened periosteum of the superior pubic ramus and medially, filling the angle between the two is the pectineal part of the inguinal ligament. Laterally is the femoral vein.

207 A hernia is an abnormal protrusion of an organ or other contents of a body compartment through the wall which normally contains them.

208 A hernia is more likely to strangulate if the neck is small and has unyielding boundaries.

209 Indirect and direct inguinal, and femoral herniae.

210 The direct hernia comes through a diffuse weakness in the abdominal wall—in that sense its route is direct. The indirect hernia traverses the inguinal canal and has an oblique or indirect route.

211 Inguinal herniae are commoner than femoral and represent about 95 per cent in men and 80 per cent in women. Of inguinal herniae the majority are indirect.

212 Inguinal hernia is the commonest inguinoscrotal swelling. This must be differentiated from the 'juvenile' hydrocele which transilluminates and in which there is no cough impulse.

213 The indirect hernia passes into the preformed sac which is an unobliterated processus vaginalis and therefore can be regarded as basically a congenital abnormality. The direct hernia is through an area of abdominal wall weakness which is acquired.

214 Femoral hernia is bilateral in 20 per cent, indirect inguinal hernia in 30 per cent and direct hernia in 50 per cent of cases.

215 An indirect inguinal hernia.

216 Epigastric hernia occurs between the recti, through the linea alba above the umbilicus. A more diffuse bulge in the midline may be due to divarication of the recti. Umbilical hernia occurs in infants while the adult hernia is usually para-umbilical. Any abdominal incision may be the site of an incisional hernia. Obturator hernia occurs through the obturator foramen and is usually very difficult to detect clinically. Rarer herniae include the Spigelian hernia (which emerges just lateral to the rectus muscle) and the lumbar hernia (which protrudes through a small defect bounded by the iliac crest, the external oblique and the latissimus dorsi muscles).

217 Exomphalos is a congenital abnormality in which the mid-gut fails to return to the coelomic cavity during intra-uterine life and remains at birth as a large hernia.

218 More than 90 per cent disappear before the baby is a year old.

219 An incisional hernia is due to disruption of the deeper layers of a laparotomy wound usually in the early postoperative period. The abdominal contents are retained only by the skin sutures and bulge later as a

hernia. Infection or poor technique may be responsible. Modern methods of mass closure or early recognition and resuture of deep dehiscence may prevent herniation later.

220 This term implies the simple transfixion of the neck and excision of the sac as opposed to any form of repair or reinforcement of the associated anatomy which would constitute herniorrhaphy.

221 After excision of the sac the anatomy is repaired so as to prevent recurrence. In the case of inguinal hernia the internal ring is narrowed and the weak posterior wall of the canal is reinforced. Various techniques have been described but darning with a monofilament suture has the advantages of avoiding tension and using a permanent but inert material for the repair.

222 When a viscus is not lying within the sac but has slid down retroperitoneally and forms the posterior wall, this is called a sliding hernia. The viscus involved is typically the caecum on the right and the sigmoid colon on the left. Sometimes the term hernia-en-glissade is used.

223 When the anatomy is very attenuated making sound repair difficult, division of the cord and orchidectomy allows the surgeon to reinforce the posterior wall more securely. Full explanation and discussion with the patient is essential whenever the possibility is anticipated and it should only be considered in older patients.

224 No. The overall recurrence rate is probably of the order of 10 per cent with most recurrences being evident within a year. Direct herniae recur more frequently than indirect.

225 After dissection the neck of the sac the abdominal wall can be resutured in overlapping layers or the defect closed by inversion of the sac and its contents. The chance of recurrence is high especially if the hernia occurred in the first place due to poor tissues. Sometimes a repair with a patch of synthetic material is necessary if the tissues are deficient.

226 Strangulation means that the hernial contents have become constricted, usually at the neck of the sac, so that the flow of blood is impaired. The veins are obstructed first and the hernial contents become engorged. As pressure builds up the inflow of arterial blood is prevented and the contents are at risk of ischaemic necrosis.

227 The risk of strangulation is highest in femoral hernia and is greater in indirect than direct inguinal hernia. The anatomy of the neck is responsible for these differences.

228 Femoral herniae are particularly liable to strangulate and may go unrecognized even after the onset of complications. Strangulation is particularly likely because of the nature of its neck, while the tendency to go unrecognized is a consequence of its usually small size and its occurrence in fat, old ladies.

229 Richter's hernia, usually femoral, contains a knuckle of strangulated bowel, but the lumen remains unobstructed as not all the circumference is involved. Littré's hernia contains a Meckel's diverticulum. Maydl's hernia or 'hernia-in-W' contains two loops of bowel and it is the intervening loop hidden inside the abdomen that is strangulated.

230 When the contents do not include the full circumference of a loop of bowel there may be strangulation without obstruction. The ischaemic contents may be omentum or only part of the bowel wall as in Richter's hernia.

231 If operation is regarded as too dangerous or if the patient refuses it is possible to manage an inguinal hernia with a truss. However, hernia repair can be performed with local or regional anaesthesia and there is rarely an absolute contra-indication to surgery.

232 If the strangulated contents include bowel its ischaemic wall will rupture in due course releasing its contents into the sac. Gangrene around the neck allows leakage into the abdominal cavity and generalized faecal peritonitis ensues. A strangulated omentocele usually remains a local problem and may develop into an abscess in the groin or scrotum.

Alimentary tract

The mouth and salivary glands

233 She has oral candidiasis, otherwise known as thrush. This is a fungal infection, due to *Candida albicans*. It is best treated with nystatin or amphotericin lozenges, continued for at least 48 hours after disappearance of the lesions. This infection is sometimes a sequel to broad spectrum antibiotic therapy, and withdrawal of such treatment should be considered if candidiasis develops.

234 At first, besides its presence on self-examination, cancer of the tongue may cause the patient no symptoms. Later, pain develops, both locally and perhaps referred to the ear. There may be excessive salivation, bleeding, reduced movement causing dysphagia and dysphonia, marked halitosis and, if lymphatic spread has occurred, a lump in the neck. On examination, the lesion usually has the typical features of a squamous cell carcinoma—a very firm ulcer with a rolled edge; alternative appearances include a warty outgrowth and an ill-defined indurated mass in the tongue.

235 The only proven pre-malignant condition is leukoplakia. Factors said to predispose to this, or directly to carcinoma, include smoking, syphilis, poor oral hygiene, malnutrition, spicy foods and alcoholism. There is no definite proof that these cause oral cancer, but they are, at least, commonly associated factors.

236 This is a soft cystic swelling in the floor of the mouth, and is in fact a mucus retention cyst. The lesion is usually globular, and can be dealt with by complete excision or wide marsupialization; sometimes, however, it extends downwards into the neck, where it can be palpated. This is known as a 'plunging ranula', requiring removal by a cervical approach.

237 He has probably developed suppurative parotitis. One or both parotid glands become the site of acute suppurative infection due to dehydration and poor oral hygiene, leading to blockage of the parotid duct with debris, and infection in the obstructed gland. It was much more common when postoperative care, in particular fluid replacement, was less satisfactory than it is today.

238 The facial, lingual and hypoglossal nerves. During parotid surgery, the facial nerve can be damaged as it runs through the substance of the gland, in which it divides into its five branches. Division of the trunk or branches produces corresponding paralysis of one side of the face. During exposure of the submandibular gland, the mandibular branch of the facial nerve can be damaged causing ugly droop of the corner of the mouth. The lingual and hypoglossal nerves can be damaged during mobilization of this gland, causing unilateral anaesthesia and paralysis of the tongue respectively.

239 The parotid duct opens beneath a small papilla on the inside of the cheek opposite the second upper molar tooth, while the submandibular duct opens on the summit of the sublingual papilla, a few millimetres lateral to the frenulum of the tongue.

240 The parotid gland is invested in an unyielding capsule, derived from the deep cervical fascia. The capsule is incapable of much expansion, so that great pressure builds up within it as the gland swells due to acute inflammation, causing severe pain.

241 The commonest parotid tumour is variously known as a mixed parotid tumour, myo-epithelioma or pleomorphic adenoma. The first of these names was the original, and was coined because this tumour was thought to be of mixed cell origin as it appeared to contain epithelial and cartilaginous elements. The 'cartilage' has since been shown to be mucin, probably secreted by myo-epithelial cells around the acini, hence the second name. The third name, pleomorphic adenoma, describes adequately the microscopic appearances, and is the one in most common usage. This tumour is usually benign, and is best treated by superficial parotidectomy, preserving the facial nerve. This procedure is preferred to enucleation of the tumour as the latter is likely to leave islands of growth, and is also more likely to lead to operative damage to the facial nerve.

242 After superficial parotidectomy, the recurrence rate is about 5 per cent. However, after removal of recurrent tumours, they recur again in 25 per cent of cases. Two to three per cent of pleomorphic adenomas become malignant, and recurrence after removal of these tumours is about 35 per cent, and double this after treatment of recurrence.

243 Yes, but calculi are fifty times more common in the submandibular duct. The stones are usually unilateral and single, although multiple stones can form in the branch ducts.

244 This is not fully understood. They are usually composed of calcium and magnesium phosphates, like the tartar that forms on teeth. This may form around minute food particles or shed cells which find their way into the duct.

245 The stone is removed under local anaesthesia, best applied on a cotton wool pledget placed under the tongue for a few minutes. The stone is immobilized by holding the soft tissues near it with forceps, and the duct opened at the site of the stone, allowing it to escape. No suture is required.

The oesophagus

246 The most important factor is the presence of a short segment of intra-abdominal oesophagus, which is kept

closed by positive intra-abdominal pressure. Other factors are the 'flap-valve' effect of the oesophagogastric angle; the high pressure zone in the lower oesophagus, in which there appears to be a physiologically active sphincter mechanism; the rosette-like folds of gastric mucosa plugging the cardia; and the right crus of the diaphragm encircling the oesophageal hiatus.

247 The oesophagus is lined throughout by stratified, non-keratinizing squamous epithelium. Deep to this is a wide submucosal layer, containing mucous glands; the muscle layer is made up of circular and longitudinal layers, which are striated in the upper third, smooth in the lower third and mixed in the middle. Between the muscle layers is the myenteric nerve plexus.

248 Dysphagia means difficulty in swallowing. The most important and common causes are carcinoma of the oesophagus, benign peptic stricture due to hiatal hernia, and achalasia of the cardia. Other causes include mediastinal malignancy, such as secondary lung cancer, retrosternal goitre, a large pharyngeal pouch, scleroderma, and neurological conditions such as bulbar palsy and myasthenia gravis.

249 Vomiting implies the expulsion of gastric contents through the mouth, while in regurgitation, food and saliva which have not reached the stomach are returned—this symptom occurs in obstructive oesophageal disease. The symptoms are differentiated by the fact that vomitus normally tastes bitter due to the admixture of gastric acid and bile, whereas regurgitated material simply has the characteristics of masticated food.

250 Potassium tablets in prolonged contact with mucosa anywhere in the alimentary tract will cause ulceration and fibrosis due to the effect of a high local concentration of potassium. Patients with cardiac disease are at particular risk, as enlargement of the left atrium causes pressure on the mid-oesophagus, so that tablets containing potassium may be held up at this level, perhaps producing an oesophageal stricture.

251 This is a squamous cell lesion, more common in men than women, and with a peak age incidence between 65 and 75 years. It causes 2500 deaths in the UK each year. Eighty per cent of growths occur in the lower half of the oesophagus. This tumour spreads locally via the submucosal layer, so that the mucosal and external appearance of the oesophagus may give a false impression of the extent of the disease. Lymphatic

spread occurs early to nodes in the neck, lung hilum or coeliac group, depending on the site of the primary. Distant, blood-borne spread is not a major feature as patients frequently die before this can occur.

252 Carcinoma of the oesophagus may be treated radically by surgical excision or radiotherapy, or palliatively by by-pass, intubation or radiotherapy. Radical surgery is only worthwhile if there is minimal spread outside the oesophagus. Radical radiotherapy has been found by some to produce good long term results and has the advantage of no operative mortality. If the growth is advanced, palliation of dysphagia is usually possible using a plastic tube passed through the lesion into the stomach.

253 This is a particularly nasty disease, as the poor prognosis illustrates—only 50 to 60 per cent are suitable for radical surgery, and in these the two year survival is only around 25 per cent.

254 Heartburn is a burning discomfort in the chest sometimes radiating to the back or neck, usually occurring after meals, on straining or on lying down. It is caused by reflux of gastric contents into the oesophagus, and is a major symptom in hiatal hernia.

255 The commonest type is the sliding hernia, in which the cardia moves up into the chest, with a variable portion of the stomach. The less common varieties are the para-oesophageal, or rolling, hernia in which the fundus of the stomach enters the chest while the cardia remains in place, and the mixed type, a combination of the sliding and rolling varieties. Most hiatal herniae are asymptomatic. Sliding hernia may present with symptoms due to gastro-oesophageal reflux, that is, heartburn and flatulence. Rolling hernia does not cause reflux but may produce anaemia due to gastric ulcer in the herniated stomach, while sometimes the latter becomes obstructed or strangulated, indicated by chest or upper abdominal pain and shock.

256 Such patients may develop peptic oesophagitis, due to acid reflux, and in a proportion of patients going on to produce ulceration, fibrosis and stricture, always at the junction of gastric and oesophageal mucosa. Refluxed material can spill over into the larynx, sometimes leading to aspiration pneumonia. Finally, some believe that carcinoma can arise at the cardia in patients with hiatal hernia.

257 The great majority of patients are helped by medical measures, aimed at minimizing reflux and reducing the effect of gastric juice on the oesophageal mucosa. Correction of obesity and cessation of smoking are

important factors. Patients should be encouraged not to stoop or strain unnecessarily and to sleep with the head of the bed raised. Medications include cimetidine, to reduce the acidity of refluxed juice; alginates, which float as a froth in the stomach, reducing reflux, and which also coat the oesophageal mucosa; and simple antacids. Surgery is indicated only if medical treatment fails after at least six months, or if complications (stenosis, bleeding, aspiration pneumonia) ensue.

258   Achalasia is a condition in which the cardia fails to relax as a bolus of food approaches, and is due to absence or paucity of ganglion cells in the myenteric plexus. The condition usually presents at the age of 20 to 40, and the typical symptoms are painless dysphagia for both solids and liquids, and a sensation of food sticking behind the lower sternum. The patient has to eat slowly, perhaps using Valsalva's manoeuvre to empty the oesophagus forcibly into the stomach. There is often a history of frequent regurgitation, sometimes with choking, and evidence of aspiration pneumonia. Barium swallow shows a greatly dilated, cucumber-shaped oesophagus, with no normal movements. Treatment is surgical—Heller's operation is performed in which the muscle, but not the mucosa, of the distal oesophagus is incised longitudinally through either an abdominal or a thoracic approach.

259   The site depends on the aetiology. The commonest benign stricture is due to acid/peptic reflux in hiatal hernia, and occurs at the junction of oesophageal and gastric mucosa, that is, usually in the distal third. Strictures due to ingestion of strong acid or alkali are often multiple, while 'potassium stricture' in cardiac patients is in the mid zone where the enlarged left atrium presses on the oesophagus. Treatment of peptic stricture is normally conservative initially, with cimetidine and dilatation of the stricture endoscopically. If this is unsuccessful, surgery for the hiatal hernia, and occasionally resection of the stricture, is required.

260   This emergency is usually first dealt with by the insertion of a Sengstaken-Blakemore tube, which applies local pressure to the oesophageal varices and their feeding veins in the gastric fundus. An alternative initial procedure is the intravenous injection of Pitressin. After initial control, endoscopic injection sclerotherapy is effective in preventing early rebleeding. More invasive measures include transabdominal devascularization of the gastric fundus, with staple-gun division and anastomosis of the lower oesophagus; transthoracic underrunning of the varices; and portasystemic shunting.

The stomach

261 Any of the structures related to the stomach can become involved with gastric cancer by direct spread. Anteriorly or above, the liver, biliary tree, abdominal wall, oesophagus and diaphragm may be invaded, while behind lie the pancreas, transverse mesocolon, spleen and posterior abdominal wall. Inferior spread can affect the transverse colon. Direct spread into several of these organs produces characteristic features. For instance, oesophageal involvement causes dysphagia, while invasion of the transverse colon may produce a gastrocolic fistula and hence the vomiting of faeces. Posterior spread into the pancreas or posterior wall musculature can produce severe back pain, so that this is a sinister symptom in a case of suspected gastric cancer.

262 The stomach has a copious arterial supply via four main arteries, the left and right gastrics, and the left and right gastro-epiploics. The left gastric artery is the largest of these; it arises directly from the coeliac axis, and passes to the upper lesser curve where it divides into superior and inferior branches. The right gastric artery usually arises from the common hepatic artery or one of its major branches and reaches the lower lesser curve near the upper border of the pylorus. The left gastro-epiploic artery arises from the splenic artery in the splenic hilum, and runs down the greater curve of the stomach to anastomose with the right gastro-epiploic artery which arises from the gastroduodenal artery near the inferior border of the pylorus. Besides these four major vessels, several short gastric arteries arise from the splenic artery at the splenic hilum to supply the upper greater curve. All these vessels give many anterior and posterior branches which anastomose profusely within the wall of the stomach. Veins corresponding to each of these arteries drain into the portal system.

263 Gastrin is produced by the G-cells in the gastric antrum. Hydrochloric acid is secreted by the parietal cells in the mucosa of the body of the stomach. Pepsin is not produced as such by the gastric mucosa— pepsinogen is secreted by the zymogen cells of the body of the stomach and converted to pepsin by the action of acid in the gastric lumen.

264 The stomach has two main functions—acid/peptic digestion of food, and temporary storage of partly digested food prior to its discharge into the duodenum for further digestion. In addition it produces intrinsic factor which binds vitamin B_{12}, ready for absorption in the distal ileum.

265 Gastric acid secretion is induced by the thought and taste of food, which cause vagal stimulation of the stomach; by the entry of food into the stomach, causing gastrin release from the antrum; and by the entry of food and its digestive products into the small bowel, acting by release of intestinal gastrins.

266 Gastric acid secretion can be reduced by drugs or by surgery. Cimetidine and ranitidine, both H2 receptor antagonists, act by blocking histamine induction of acid release, the final common pathway for all modes of gastric acid secretion. This approach has been a major step forward in the medical treatment of peptic ulcer disease. Surgical methods of reducing gastric acid secretion are vagotomy in its various forms; antrectomy, which removes the gastrin-producing area of the stomach; and total gastrectomy, which removes the acid-producing area, as well as the antrum, and is the only procedure which can totally abolish acid production.

267 Gastric cancer usually develops insidiously, so that it is usually advanced by the time of diagnosis. Most patients give a story of persistent indigestion with anorexia and weight loss. The patient is often anaemic and may have an epigastric mass. Sometimes the lesion will cause dysphagia at an early stage, due to involvement of the cardio-oesophageal junction, while in a minority haematemesis or perforation will be the mode of presentation. In a few, spread beyond the stomach will lead to ascites due to peritoneal spread; jaundice due to liver secondaries; or a lump in the neck due to lymphatic spread (Troisier's sign).

268 Gastric cancer arises more frequently in patients with pernicious anaemia or who have undergone partial gastrectomy for peptic ulcer. It is apparent that gastric cancer may arise from areas of intestinal metaplasia within the stomach, and that, in the rare instance when true adenomas are present in the stomach, these may become malignant.

269 Otherwise known as leather-bottle stomach, this is a form of gastric cancer in which the tumour not only spreads widely in the submucosa and muscularis, but also excites an extensive fibrotic reaction which converts the stomach into a thick, narrow, rigid tube. There is usually no focal mucosal lesion to be seen. It represents about seven per cent of all cases of gastric cancer, and carries the worst prognosis of all forms.

270 Operations for gastric cancer may be radical or palliative. Radical operations, performed in the hope of cure, involve removal of all or most of the stomach,

together with its lymphatic drainage and any locally involved adjacent tissue, followed by a reconstruction to restore continuity. Palliative surgery may amount to removal of the primary—as a subtotal gastrectomy—in cases where distant spread has rendered the patient incurable; sometimes the tumour is irremovably invading locally, so that a gastrojejunostomy bypassing the growth is all that is possible. Radical surgery is feasible in about 50 per cent of cases and palliative surgery in 20 per cent, while in the remainder the growth is beyond any surgical help at the time of laparotomy.

271 In general, no—the median survival of all cases is less than six months. About 10 per cent of all patients survive for five years, and even if radical resection has been possible, the corresponding figure is only about 30 per cent. The only group of patients with a good prognosis are those with the lesion called 'early gastric cancer' in which the tumour is confined to the mucosa and submucosa, with or without lymphatic involvement—in this group the five-year survival is at least 70 per cent after radical surgery.

272 Weight loss in gastric ulcer patients is common due to the tendency for them to avoid eating for fear of bringing on their pain. However, the possibility must be borne in mind that the ulcer might be a malignancy, and that this may be the cause of the weight loss.

273 Back pain in such a patient suggests penetration of the ulcer through the posterior wall of the stomach, into structures in the stomach bed, usually the pancreas. Penetration can occur with benign or malignant ulcers, so back pain does not necessarily indicate carcinoma.

274 Unlike duodenal ulcer, gastric ulcers are sometimes malignant—clinical and radiological evidence alone cannot exclude carcinoma. Therefore, before beginning a trial of medical treatment for any gastric ulcer, endoscopy should be carried out to allow careful, direct inspection of the lesion and, more importantly, multiple biopsy of the edge and base of the ulcer.

275 Assuming that the ulcer has been carefully investigated by x-ray, endoscopy and multiple biopsy, it is safe to try to heal it by medical means. The patient should first be told to stop smoking and to take a regular diet. Medication may take various forms—in particular cimetidine may be prescribed to decrease acid secretion, and carbenoxolone or bismuth compounds may be used to aid the protection of the mucosa, either by an effect on the gastric mucus or

directly. If the ulcer has not healed within 8 to 12 weeks, or if complications supervene, operation should be advised.

276 There are three, possibly four, complications of gastric ulcer; haemorrhage, perforation, stenosis of the stomach at the level of the ulcer, and malignant change. The last of these is questionable as a complication of benign ulcer—some would say that 'ulcer cancers' are malignant from the outset.

277 The features of a gastric ulcer that should be checked when deciding whether it might be malignant are its site and its profile. While ulcers sited on the lesser curve can be benign or malignant, ulcers elsewhere in the stomach should be viewed with particular suspicion. If the ulcer is shown in profile, one should check whether the base lies outside the contour of the stomach, or within it suggesting ulceration of a cancer encroaching on the lumen. However, neither of these signs is sufficiently specific, so that endoscopy and biopsy remain necessary.

278 This is a condition in which multiple shallow ulcers, usually less than 5 mm in diameter, develop in the stomach. There may be a few, or the whole mucosa may be affected. The intervening mucosa is often oedematous and engorged, and there may be areas of submucosal haemorrhage. This condition usually develops in patients very ill from some other problem, and is often encountered in the Intensive Care Unit. Patients with severe burns, head injuries, strokes, overwhelming sepsis, respiratory, renal or liver failure are all prone to erosive gastritis. It can also occur in alcohol abuse, or after the use of aspirin and other anti-inflammatory drugs.

279 The major element of the management of a case of bleeding erosive gastritis is circulatory support—the bleeding is usually not severe and can be expected to stop spontaneously in most cases. Blood loss is replaced; cimetidine is usually given intravenously, though there is little evidence of its positive value in this situation. If bleeding continues, vasopressin may be given, while therapeutic embolization may be considered if this fails. Surgery is the last resort, as it is often ineffective in this condition, and carries a high mortality; if surgery is necessary, vagotomy with partial gastrectomy is probably the procedure of choice.

280 The commonest causes of upper gastro-intestinal haemorrhage are duodenal ulcer, gastric ulcer and acute gastric erosions—these lesions account for more

than 80 per cent of cases. Mallory-Weiss mucosal tears at the cardia, oesophageal varices and gastric neoplasms account for most of the remainder.

281 Early endoscopy is popular among clinicians treating upper gastro-intestinal haemorrhage because it provides a definitive diagnosis in most cases, allowing treatment to be more precisely tailored to the underlying cause. In particular, it picks out those patients in whom bleeding is unlikely to respond to resuscitation alone (oesophageal varices) and vice versa (gastric erosions). However, as yet there is no convincing evidence that this apparently useful tool sufficiently improves management that it reduces overall mortality in upper GI bleeding.

282 The operations available for bleeding peptic ulcer range from simple underrunning of the bleeding vessel, through vagotomy and pyloroplasty, to partial gastrectomy. Most surgeons would agree that simple suture is not enough except in the most extreme circumstances. Partial gastrectomy, either Billroth 1 for gastric ulcer or Polya for duodenal ulcer, has the advantages of removing the ulcer as well as decreasing acid production, and has low incidence of recurrent, potentially lethal, problems—however, the operation may be technically difficult. On balance, many surgeons would opt for partial gastrectomy in the average case that comes to surgery for bleeding peptic ulcer.

283 The overall mortality is about 10 per cent and this figure has not changed in several decades, despite better general care, and the use of emergency endoscopy; however, the average age has increased, offsetting an improved outlook in younger patients. Lesions with a worse than average prognosis are bleeding chronic gastric ulcer and oesophageal varices.

The duodenum

284 The duodenal cap is the first part of the duodenum— this is a term used mainly by radiologists, who see it as a triangular area with rounded corners on barium meal examination.

285 By convention, the term 'penetration' implies the extension of peptic ulceration through the posterior wall, as opposed to anterior perforation into the peritoneal cavity. Therefore the structures lying behind the first part of the duodenum may be penetrated—these are the gastroduodenal artery and its branches, which may bleed, and the pancreas, causing back pain.

286 The duodenal mucosa secretes cholecystokinin-pancreozymin, secretin and enterogastrone. All three are released into the portal vein when the initial products of digestion leave the stomach. CCK-PZ stimulates the gall bladder to contract and the pancreas to secrete enzymes into the pancreatic juice; secretin stimulates the pancreas to release water and electrolytes into the duct system; while enterogastrone inhibits gastric secretion and motility, probably by inhibiting gastrin release.

287 There are two protective mechanisms—the mucus barrier and neutralization of acid by the alkaline bile and pancreatic juice; secretion of both is stimulated by the passage of acid gastric content into the duodenum.

288 The usual symptoms of duodenal ulcer are epigastric pain which comes on several hours after meals, that is, prior to the next meal, which is relieved by food or alkalis, and which may also wake the patient in the early hours, when again it is relieved by nourishment. These symptoms are usually periodic, troubling the patient for a month or two, followed by a remission of similar length. The patient is more often male than female, aged 25 to 50, probably smokes, and is likely to have a stressful existence, either because of his personality or his job.

289 Water brash is the sudden filling of the mouth with 'water' (saliva), and is sometimes encountered in patients with duodenal ulcer.

290 In a patient with the appropriate symptoms, barium meal examination is usually sufficient to confirm the diagnosis—the duodenum will appear deformed due to scarring, and there will be a central spot of barium indicating the ulcer crater. Endoscopy is usually not necessary, except when the clinical and radiological findings are in doubt; biopsy is never required as duodenal ulcer is never malignant.

291 The patient should be told to stop smoking and lead a more ordered existence. The treatment of choice today is a histamine H2-receptor antagonist, either cimetidine or ranitidine, which will induce a major decrease in gastric acid output. Symptoms are usually rapidly relieved, and the ulcer heals soon afterwards. However, treatment must continue indefinitely as it does not cure the disease, just suppresses it.

292 Medical management can be said to have failed if it has not reduced symptoms to a point at which the patient can live his normal life comfortably (this is usually reflected in his ability to go to work regularly),

or if, despite medical therapy, complications supervene.

293   Surgery is indicated in duodenal ulcer if medical management fails to produce adequate symptomatic relief, or if any of the complications arise (perforation, major haemorrhage, or pyloric stenosis).

294   Nowadays, most surgeons perform some form of vagotomy for duodenal ulcer—this may be a truncal or selective vagotomy with either a pyloroplasty or gastro-enterostomy, or a highly selective vagotomy without a drainage procedure. In some circumstances, particularly when a duodenal ulcer is bleeding, a partial gastrectomy may be appropriate. Some surgeons combine the two types of operation by performing vagotomy and antrectomy, which has the lowest rate of ulcer recurrence.

295   Highly selective vagotomy involves division of the branches supplying the parietal cells of the stomach (thus decreasing acid secretion), while sparing the branches to the antrum (thus maintaining normal gastric motility). Therefore, although a pyloroplasty or gastro-enterostomy is normally performed with a truncal or selective vagotomy, which paralyse the stomach, this is not required with a highly selective vagotomy.

296   The main long-term complications are recurrent ulcer and diarrhoea, both more common after vagotomy than gastrectomy; dumping, anaemia, bilious vomiting and gastric cancer are more common after gastrectomy than vagotomy.

The pancreas

297   The pancreas has an autonomic nerve supply, both sympathetic and parasympathetic, arising from the coeliac plexus, around the origin of the coeliac artery. This assumes clinical importance in patients with pancreatic cancer, in whom percutaneous destruction of the coeliac plexus, using injections of alcohol or phenol, may be used for pain relief.

298   The major factors in the promotion of pancreatic exocrine secretion are the hormones secretin and cholecystokinin-pancreozymin. They are released into the portal blood by duodenal and upper small bowel mucosa when acid and initial products of digestion leave the stomach. Secretin promotes water and electrolyte secretion, while CCK-PZ promotes enzyme

release into pancreatic juice. As gastric emptying
ceases, hormone drive on the pancreas diminishes, so
that secretion is inhibited.

299 While the classical triad of weight loss, jaundice and
pain can occur in any case of pancreatic cancer,
jaundice is more frequent when the growth is in the
head, and pain is more common in body or tail lesions.
Lesions in the head often involve the bile duct, so
jaundice is present on first visit in 80 per cent; in more
distal lesions, jaundice does not develop until there are
liver metastases. Pain is less common at initial
presentation in head lesions because jaundice develops
early, leading to earlier presentation compared to body
and tail growths, which have frequently spread into
the posterior abdominal wall when first seen.

300 Extra-abdominal manifestations of pancreatic cancer,
which occur with varying frequency, include
supraclavicular lymph node involvement; thrombotic
episodes, either spontaneous DVT, or thrombophlebitis
migrans in which thromboses occur repeatedly in
different peripheral sites; acanthosis nigricans, a dark,
raised skin lesion, usually occurring in the axillae; and
psychiatric disturbances, which may precede somatic
symptoms.

301 Sometimes. As with any tumour, proof depends on
acquiring tissue diagnosis. In pancreatic cancer,
cytological specimens may be recovered by endoscopic
brushing or collection of pancreatic juice, or by
ultrasound-directed percutaneous needle aspiration of
the lesion. Other diagnostic methods, including
various radiological approaches, can only provide
suggestive evidence.

302 Cancer of the pancreas is the least curable of
intra-abdominal malignancies. Only rarely is the
lesion small enough to warrant an attempt at radical
surgery—it must be no larger than 2 cm and must be
confined to the pancreas—and even then the five-year
survival is low. All other patients can only be
palliated; this includes by-pass surgery for biliary or
duodenal obstruction, and coeliac plexus block to deal
with pain.

303 This term should be used only in patients with
pancreatic pain and with evidence of pancreatic
exocrine insufficiency in whom the pancreas has been
shown radiologically or at operation to be the site of
disease. It may be complicated by recurrent episodes of
acute pancreatitis. The pathological process is
progressive, irreversible inflammation, usually caused
by alcohol or by gallstone disease. Initially there is

plugging of minor ducts causing dilatation and fibrosis, the process later spreading to the major ducts.

304 Patients suffering from chronic pancreatitis require a high protein, high calorie diet, and must stop drinking. Further treatment depends on symptoms— malabsorption can be treated with pancreatic enzyme replacement tablets, and diabetes is managed appropriately. If pain or jaundice are the main problems, surgery must be considered. ERCP should be performed to determine the anatomy of the diseased pancreas and the state of the bile duct. Surgery aims at decompressing the obstructed pancreatic duct, usually by distal resection and drainage into the small bowel, or by longitudinal pancreatojejunostomy.

305 This is a collection of pancreatic secretion and inflammatory exudate in the lesser sac in some cases of acute or chronic pancreatitis, which may be responsible for continued discomfort and debility; it is lined by fibrous and inflammatory tissue rather than epithelium—hence the term 'pseudocyst'. Its presence may be suspected from the history and a mass in the epigastrium, while confirmation is usually obtained by ultrasound examination. Some pseudocysts resolve spontaneously but the larger, symptomatic ones require surgery. The cyst is approached through the stomach, a wide opening being made into the cyst through the posterior wall—cystogastrostomy. The cyst contents drain into the stomach, after which the opening in the stomach closes spontaneously.

The liver

306 The dividing line between the functional lobes of the liver runs along the plane lying vertically through the bed of the gall bladder anteriorly and the vena cava behind; this differs from the old anatomical division, which lies further to the left, in the plane of the falciform ligament. The functional division is important during resection of a liver lobe, as it is the plane marking the watershed between the territories of the right and left hepatic arteries, and hence must be followed to avoid major haemorrhage.

307 During the usual lateral approach, the lung may be punctured if the patient has not breathed out fully. The gall bladder, the structures in the free edge of the lesser omentum, the duodenum and the hepatic flexure of the colon can all be damaged if the needle is pushed in too far, and especially if an anterior approach is used. The kidney may also be injured.

308   Liver secondaries can be suspected clinically if the liver is enlarged and irregular; they can be seen at operation; they can be detected by ultrasound, isotope scanning or CT scan; but they can be proven only on histological examination of material taken by needle biopsy or at operation. Changes in blood tests, particularly the serum alkaline phosphatase and bilirubin, occur only when there is massive replacement of liver tissue by secondary deposits and are thus a late indicator.

309   It is sometimes possible to remove solitary secondaries curatively, while multiple, symptomatic deposits are sometimes amenable to palliative treatment. Curative resection should only be attempted for colorectal secondaries, and then only if investigations suggest that the disease is localized to one lobe, in which case a wedge or even a lobe can be resected. There is no prospect of cure with other primary sites. Palliation of pain due to secondaries from any site can sometimes be achieved by the radiologist using embolization via an arterial catheter.

310   The most common predisposing factor is cirrhosis, especially when induced by alcohol or hepatitis B. Very important factors elsewhere in the world are aflatoxin contamination of food in Southern Africa, and liver fluke infestation in the Far East.

311   Hydatid disease—infestation with *Echinococcus granulosus*. This organism is ingested by humans via the faecal-oral route from dogs which excrete the eggs, having eaten offal from sheep already infested with *Echinococcus*. The organisms travel via the portal system to the liver, where they form cysts, inside which smaller daughter cysts proliferate. Other organs, particularly the lung, can become infested.

312   Amoebiasis. This is caused by the protozoan *Entamoeba histolytica*, and is primarily a disease of the colon; sometimes the organism reaches the liver to produce an amoebic abscess. This lesion is usually treated by a combination of aspiration and either metronidazole or tinidazole by mouth, though sometimes open drainage or the use of the older drugs, particularly emetine, is required.

313   Liver abscesses in Britain are almost always pyogenic, and occur most frequently in patients with biliary disease or some form of pre-existing malignancy or an inflammatory condition such as diverticular disease.

314   The two essentials in the treatment of unilocular liver abscess are drainage and adequate antibiotics. Drainage may be by closed aspiration via a tube

inserted with ultrasound or CT guidance, or by open operation. Antibiotics should initially be a wide spectrum combination, such as tobramycin, ampicillin and metronidazole, until examination of the pus allows a more specific approach.

315 Oesophageal varices are thin-walled veins in the submucosa of the oesophagus, occurring in patients with portal hypertension, and constituting abnormal portasystemic communications via which the portal system decompresses into the systemic venous system. They are of particular importance as they are liable to rupture, causing torrential haemorrhage.

The biliary tree

316 The structures in greatest danger are the extrahepatic biliary tree and the blood vessels supplying the liver. Damage may occur if an adequate view of the various structures is not ensured during dissection—this may be hampered by the build of the patient, poor lighting and inadequate assistance. If unexpected bleeding occurs, blind attempts to stop it can lead to accidental duct injuries. Less commonly, anatomical anomalies lead to mistaken ligation and division of vital ducts or vessels.

317 The distal common bile duct passes behind the pancreas to enter the duodenum, usually in its second part, at the papilla of Vater. As the duct passes through the duodenal wall it is surrounded by a cuff of muscle of variable length, the sphincter of Oddi. In about 75 per cent of individuals the pancreatic duct enters the distal common duct through the sphincter of Oddi; in the remainder it either enters the duct above the sphincter, or enters the duodenum separately.

318 Bile is unique in being both an exocrine secretion, playing a role in digestion, and a major excretory pathway. The digestive function is played by bile acids and phospholipids, which form micelles or 'packets' of water-insoluble dietary lipids, ready for absorption; in addition bile acids activate pancreatic lipase. Bile contains excreted bilirubin and cholesterol, the latter held in solution by micelle formation with the bile acids and phospholipids.

319 It appears that most gallstones develop due to changes in the relative proportions of bile acids, phospholipids and cholesterol in the bile. As the latter, which is water insoluble, is held in solution by aggregation with the other two constituents, increase in cholesterol content or decrease in bile acid content lead to cholesterol microcrystal formation and later to

gall-stones. Increased cholesterol content occurs in people on the contraceptive pill or on clofibrate, and may also be related to a highly refined Western diet. Bile acid concentration may fall in patients with abnormal enterohepatic circulation, such as those with Crohn's disease or a small bowel fistula. Pigment stones are common in patients with chronic haemolytic disease (in whom bile pigment excretion is excessive) such as sickle-cell anaemia.

320 Gallstones are commonest in middle-aged, overweight mothers. Typically, the patient complains of postprandial discomfort sometimes amounting to pain, in the epigastrium or right upper quadrant which may radiate to the right scapular area. Symptoms may be especially bad after fatty or fried foods. If gallstones are confirmed in these people, they are said to be suffering from chronic cholecystitis.

321 Besides chronic cholecystitis, gallstones may declare themselves by causing acute cholecystitis, biliary colic, or obstructive jaundice. Much less commonly they present as empyema of the gall bladder, ascending cholangitis, or gallstone ileus.

322 In the majority of patients the diagnosis is confirmed by oral cholecystography. This is a two-day radiological procedure. Plain films are taken one day, the patient takes tablets containing an iodine compound that night and further films are taken the next day as the contrast is concentrated in the gall bladder, if it is functioning. A simpler technique is biliary ultrasonography. This not only allows confirmation of stones in the gall bladder but also provides information about the bile duct and pancreas, and can be used in jaundiced patients. This technique is more liable to error in interpretation of results, and hence sometimes less reliable. Another technique sometimes used in acutely ill or jaundiced patients is HIDA scanning, an intravenous isotope technique in which a radiolabelled substance is rapidly excreted into the bile allowing biliary imaging—'absence' of a gall bladder arising from the bile duct suggests cystic duct obstruction.

323 Those suffering from biliary colic are cured by cholecystectomy, while patients with 'chronic cholecystitis' (postprandial discomfort, fatty food intolerance, etc.), although spared the chance of later gallstone complications, may continue to suffer their dyspeptic symptoms, and are therefore the group least helped by cholecystectomy.

324 After adequate exposure via a paramedian or subcostal incision, and inspection of all abdominal contents, a

careful dissection is made to expose Calot's triangle, in particular the cystic duct and artery. The cystic artery is tied and divided, followed by intubation of the cystic duct to allow operative cholangiography; having thus confirmed the anatomy and excluded common duct stones, the cystic duct is divided and tied, and the gall bladder stripped from its fossa. After careful haemostasis a drain is placed in the subhepatic space, and the abdomen closed.

325 This is a radiological technique which allows confirmation of the anatomy of the biliary tree prior to division of the presumed cystic duct, and demonstrates abnormalities of the extrahepatic duct such as dilatation and duct stones. It is performed by injecting contrast via a small cannula in the cystic duct, and exposing three x-ray films after repeated injections, the films being placed in a tunnel under the patient. Operative cholangiography provides a more reliable basis for the decision to explore the bile duct than is possible using clinical data and duct palpation alone, leading to fewer unproductive explorations and lower morbidity.

326 In some patients gallstones can be removed by dissolution. Stones consisting mainly of cholesterol can be made to dissolve by giving the bile acid, chenodeoxycholic acid, orally for long periods. However, this treatment has drawbacks—the gall bladder must be functioning; the stones must not contain calcium, as judged on x-ray, and they should be small; the patient should not be a young woman likely to become pregnant, and should not have liver disease or be suffering frequent bouts of biliary pain. Furthermore, the stones are very likely to recur if therapy is stopped.

327 This term implies jaundice due to mechanical obstruction of the extrahepatic biliary tree. The commonest causes of obstructive jaundice are gallstones in the bile duct, and carcinoma of the head of pancreas. Less common are carcinoma of the ampulla of Vater, or of the bile duct; traumatic duct stricture, due to previous surgery; sclerosing cholangitis; pancreatitis; and parasitic infestation of the duct. It is very important to differentiate jaundice due to one of these 'surgical' conditions from 'cholestatic' jaundice (which is caused by intrahepatic small duct obstruction due to a drug reaction, hepatitis, or cirrhosis, and which has many of the clinical and biochemical features of obstruction), as surgery in this group would be totally inappropriate.

328 This is probably due to the deposition of bile acids in the skin. Besides the use of conventional antipruritic

treatment, cholestyramine can be administered which may help by increasing faecal loss of bile acids.

329 The typical changes in liver function tests in obstructive jaundice (besides a raised bilirubin) are a markedly raised alkaline phosphatase, with lesser rises in the hepatocellular enzymes. However, a biochemically 'obstructive' picture is also found in patients with intrahepatic cholestasis due to medical causes, so chemistry alone is not sufficient to prove extrahepatic obstruction.

330 This is a radiological investigation in which contrast medium is injected into the intrahepatic biliary tree. A needle is inserted into the liver percutaneously under local anaesthetic and withdrawn until bile is aspirated, indicating that the end of the needle is in an intrahepatic bile duct. Screening following injection of contrast confirms correct placement, after which a soft cannula is passed down the needle into the biliary tree. More contrast medium is then injected to produce pictures of the intra- and extrahepatic bile ducts. If ultrasonography and ERCP are not available, this procedure is useful in confirming that a case of jaundice is due to extrahepatic obstruction, and in delineating the lesion prior to surgery. It is particularly helpful in potentially complicated operative cases, such as iatrogenic duct strictures and bile duct carcinomas, in which the operative dissection and peroperative radiology may be difficult.

331 This term refers to the renal failure which may develop in the patient undergoing surgery for obstructive jaundice. The exact cause for this problem is not clear, but it seems that the renal tubules are especially sensitive to ischaemic damage in hyperbilirubinaemia and in the endotoxaemia resulting from the poor reticulo-endothelial function of the compromised liver. Prophylaxis involves maintaining a diuresis throughout the perioperative period using a fluid load and mannitol infusion; in addition, full antibiotic cover may decrease endotoxaemia.

332 A T-tube is a drainage device used following exploration of the common bile duct; it consists of a soft rubber tube in the shape of a T, the transverse limb of which is placed in the duct while the vertical limb is brought out to the skin via a stab incision. The tube is left to drain into a bag for 10 days after surgery; if a stone has been left in the distal duct, the decompressive effect of the tube prevents leakage of bile into the peritoneum at the site of exploration. After 10 days, a T-tube cholangiogram is performed to exclude a retained stone; if all is well the tube is

clamped for 24 hours and then simply pulled out. During the postoperative period, a track will have formed around the long limb of the tube, so that any transient leak of bile following tube removal passes harmlessly to the skin surface.

333 Nowadays, the retained stone can usually be dealt with by non-operative means. Small distal stones often pass spontaneously, while others can sometimes be flushed out of the duct by T-tube injection of saline, or dissolved by slow infusion of cholic acid or heparin. If these simple measures do not work, the T-tube is left in situ for six weeks to produce a mature track around it; most stones can then be retrieved using a steerable catheter and stone basket passed down the T-tube track. If this fails, endoscopic sphincterotomy, and removal by catheter basket will cope with almost all remaining stones.

334 A mucocele of the gall bladder occurs when the organ becomes distended with mucus; it develops when a gall-stone impacts in the cystic duct or Hartmann's pouch, preventing entry of bile or exit of gall bladder mucus. If acute infection does not supervene, producing an empyema, the gall bladder mucosa will absorb the bile salts and pigments, which will be carried away in the blood stream, and replace them with mucus. The gall bladder can become greatly distended, and hence palpable below the right costal margin.

335 Bile duct strictures may be benign or malignant. More than 90 per cent of benign strictures follow surgery on the biliary tract, while the remainder are due to other upper abdominal surgery, chronic pancreatitis or sclerosing cholangitis. Bile duct carcinoma is uncommon.

336 Although an uncommon disease, this is in fact the fifth most common digestive malignancy; it usually occurs in association with gall-stones. It spreads by local invasion of the liver and other surrounding organs, and to the local lymph nodes. The diagnosis is often first made at cholecystectomy for gall-stones; the tumour is usually unresectable, so that the prognosis is dismal—80 per cent are dead at one year, with a five-year survival of less than five per cent.

The spleen

337 The organs in particular danger are the pancreas, stomach and diaphragm. The pancreatic tail lies at the splenic hilum and can be damaged during ligation of the artery and vein; the upper part of the greater curve

of the stomach is supplied by the short gastric branches of the splenic artery, so the stomach can be caught in the ties on these vessels; and the diaphragm may be adherent to the posterior surface of the spleen, in which case it can be pierced during initial mobilization. Other structures occasionally traumatized are the left kidney and adrenal gland, and the splenic flexure of the colon.

338   The signs that suggest that an abdominal mass is an enlarged spleen are as follows: first, on palpation, it is smooth, has a discrete lower border, perhaps with a notch, and its upper border is out of reach, beneath the left costal margin; second, it moves downwards on inspiration; and third, it is dull to percussion. Sometimes, if the spleen is massively enlarged, reaching to the pelvis, several of these points cannot be confirmed.

339   The commonest causes of splenomegaly in Britain are the myeloproliferative disorders, particularly myeloid leukaemia and Hodgkin's disease, portal hypertension due to cirrhosis, thrombocytopenic purpura and spherocytosis.

340   The usual indications for splenectomy are trauma, as a staging procedure in Hodgkin's disease, as a therapeutic measure in blood diseases such as thrombocytopenic purpura and spherocytosis, and to correct hypersplenism in leukaemia or cirrhosis.

341   The early complications of splenectomy include haemorrhage from the splenic pedicle or splenic bed; venous thrombosis as a result of the greatly increased platelet count which may follow splenectomy; and fistula resulting from damage to the pancreas, stomach or colon. The important late complication is overwhelming sepsis, particularly in small children.

342   These are small 'accessory spleens', often a centimetre or two in diameter, and usually located in the splenic hilum, in the gastrosplenic ligament or in the greater omentum. They are only of importance when splenectomy is performed to treat blood disease—splenunculi must always be sought in these cases, as if left, they may grow to cause recurrence of the original problem.

The small bowel

343   The superior mesenteric artery supplies the small bowel. Having arisen from the aorta behind the pancreas, it passes downwards between the uncinate process and the neck of the pancreas to cross the third

part of the duodenum, thus entering the root of the small bowel mesentery. Therein it runs downwards to the right towards its termination, about six inches proximal to the ileocaecal valve, crossing the vena cava, right psoas muscle and right ureter en route.

344 As the terminal ileum is the site of absorption of the intrinsic factor/vitamin B_{12} complex and the reabsorption of bile salts, there are two main consequences of its resection—first, megaloblastic anaemia may develop when vitamin B_{12} stores become depleted, and second, depletion of the bile salt pool can lead to diarrhoea.

345 Most patients with small bowel Crohn's disease initially present with diarrhoea, colicky abdominal pain, malaise and weight loss. On examination there may be a mild pyrexia and in about 30 per cent a mass may be felt, usually in the right iliac fossa. Around 10 per cent of patients will have anal disease, fistula or fissure, even in the absence of other evidence of large bowel involvement with Crohn's disease.

346 The most important extra-abdominal manifestation of Crohn's disease is perianal sepsis—this may take the form of anal fissure (often multiple, and with angry, oedematous surrounding skin) or fistula-in-ano, which may be complicated or accompanied by cavitation. Other such signs of Crohn's disease include oral aphthous ulceration, polyarthritis and erythema nodosum.

347 A barium follow-through examination will demonstrate several features in Crohn's disease. First, there will be one or more segments of abnormality, usually in the distal small bowel—if there are more than one, they are known as skip lesions. Abnormal segments have a narrow, irregular lumen, with a thickened wall which holds other loops of bowel away, so that the narrowed segment stands out—the string sign of Kantor. Mucosal ulceration is usually visible, and there may be evidence of fistulae into other parts of the small or large bowel, into the bladder or occasionally on to the skin.

348 Surgery is undertaken for Crohn's disease in several circumstances: first, in patients initially treated medically who fail to thrive, that is, remain unwell, underweight, anaemic and uncomfortable; second, surgery is indicated for the complications, particularly obstruction, fistula, and abscess formation; finally, it is sometimes necessary in order to contain the extra-abdominal manifestations of the disease, which usually improve once the diseased bowel is excised.

349 At operation, the features that indicate the presence of Crohn's disease are the occurrence of stiff, contracted, hyperaemic segments of small bowel—so-called 'hose-pipe' bowel—with a thickened mesentery containing enlarged lymph nodes. The mesenteric fat may encroach abnormally far around the circumference of the bowel. There may be evidence of intimate adherence of abnormal bowel to other loops, suggesting fistula formation.

350 There are four ways in which Meckel's diverticulum can induce acute illness; it can become acutely inflamed—Meckel's diverticulitis—which precisely mimics acute appendicitis; it can cause small bowel obstruction by becoming adherent somewhere within the abdomen, often due to a fibrous band at its apex; it can perforate, usually at an ulcer arising at an island of ectopic gastric mucosa within it; or it can bleed from an ectopic peptic ulcer.

351 The great majority of cases of small bowel obstruction are due to groin hernia or postoperative adhesions. A minority are due to a range of other causes including volvulus around congenital bands, loops of bowel forming stomas or gastro-enterostomies; appendicitis; small bowel tumours, both primary adenocarcinomas, and secondary ovarian and pancreatic cancer and, oddly, melanoma; impassable objects in the lumen, including foreign bodies, gallstones and boluses of indigestible food; and, very rarely, internal herniae.

352 There are three points about the fashioning of an ileostomy which deserve comment. First, its position—it is placed in the lower abdomen, away from the umbilicus, the anterior superior iliac spine, scars and the belt line so that the appliance fits nicely and is comfortable. Second, its spout shape—this is used so that the apex of the stoma lies well into the appliance to avoid skin maceration. Finally, the mucocutaneous suture—early ileostomies were simply spouts of bowel brought out through the skin, but the serosal surface often became fibrotic and contracted, leading to sub-acute obstruction. Simple doubling back of the bowel, and suture of the mucosa to the skin edge has largely overcome mechanical complications. Having an ileostomy can never be pleasant, but some cope better than others. It tends to produce liquid effluent continuously throughout the day, and may overact if there is dietary indiscretion. It needs regular and careful maintenance to prevent skin damage. However, it need not prevent a full and active working and social life.

The peritoneal cavity

353 Ascites is diagnosed clinically by finding abdominal distension, a fluid thrill and shifting dullness. The first sign is non-specific, and could otherwise be due to gaseous distension or a large mass, such as an ovarian cyst. A fluid thrill confirms the presence of a large volume of fluid, and is elicited by flicking one side of the abdomen with the index finger and feeling the transmitted thrill with the other hand on the other side of the abdomen, while the edge of an assistant's hand presses on the centre of the abdomen to prevent transmission via the abdominal wall. The fact that the fluid is free within the peritoneum rather than in a cyst is confirmed by the shifting dullness test in which the pattern of peripheral dullness and central resonance changes when the patient rolls 45 degrees sideways, so that the gas in the intestine floats uppermost again. If doubt still exists ultrasound examination can be performed. The major causes of ascites are malignancy, portal hypertension, usually due to cirrhosis, right heart failure and the nephrotic syndrome.

354 The ascites can be drained to produce short-term relief, and chemotherapeutic agents instilled to try to prevent reaccumulation. This is best done, after making sure that the bladder is empty, by inserting a peritoneal dialysis cannula into the pelvis via the right iliac fossa or the linea alba under local anaesthesia. When all the fluid is drained, thiotepa, an alkylating agent, is injected via the cannula—the dose is 10 to 30 mg in 20 to 60 ml of sterile water; this can be repeated every one or two weeks if necessary.

355 Pelvic abscess is most commonly seen in patients who have already been treated for an intraperitoneal infective process, rather than in patients presenting de novo. The important initiating lesions are perforated appendicitis, perforated peptic ulcer and perforated diverticular disease. The symptoms suggestive of this condition are pelvic discomfort and diarrhoea, while on examination there is a swinging fever, and fullness of the pouch of Douglas, with induration of the overlying rectal wall. If necessary, the diagnosis is confirmed by ultrasound. Treatment is expectant—the abscess usually drains spontaneously through the anterior rectal wall.

356 An appendix abscess is diagnosed on several criteria—the patient usually has a history, perhaps five or six days long, suggestive of appendicitis. On examination there is a right iliac fossa mass which is tender, and there is a swinging pyrexia, perhaps

associated with rigors. It is important to differentiate an abscess from a solid inflammatory mass due to appendicitis, or even to Crohn's disease, as the treatment of abscess is surgical, while a solid lesion is managed conservatively. An appendix abscess should be drained, with no attempt to remove the appendix unless it is technically easy, as attempts to locate the appendix in the abscess can lead to damage to the surrounding bowel. Appendicectomy is performed six or eight weeks later when the inflammation has settled.

The large bowel

357 The colon as far as the distal transverse colon is supplied by branches of the superior mesenteric artery, i.e., the ileocolic, right colic and middle colic arteries. The colon from the splenic flexure distally, and the rectum, are supplied by the left colic, sigmoid and superior haemorrhoidal branches of the inferior mesenteric artery. The middle rectal branch of the internal iliac artery also contributes to the supply of the rectum.

358 The main point is that the longitudinal muscle of the colon is confined to the three taeniae coli, whereas it is spread evenly around the rectum. The blood vessels of the colon penetrate the wall vertically at the edges of the taeniae, producing potential 'channels' along which intraluminal pressure can, over a period, force the development of mucosal diverticula. However, the vessels supplying the rectum penetrate the wall more obliquely, so that luminal pressure does not force out diverticula alongside them.

359 The right ureter and kidney, the right testicular or ovarian vessels, the duodenum and pancreas.

360 The large bowel absorbs water and electrolytes from the material entering it from the ileum, and acts as a reservoir for faecal matter until voiding is socially convenient. Of the 800 to 1000 ml of water presented to the large bowel each day, all but 150 ml is absorbed. Voiding of faeces is controlled by a complicated sensorimotor mechanism in which awareness of the presence of faeces in the rectum is mediated by nerve endings in the pelvic floor; when the rectum is thus distended, a reflex relaxes the anal sphincter, though this can be voluntarily overridden if the time is not right for defaecation.

361 Fifty per cent of all large bowel cancers occur in the rectum, a further 25 per cent in the sigmoid colon, and

about 10 per cent in the caecum. The remainder are spread fairly evenly throughout the rest of the colon.

362 Right-sided cancer classically presents with the symptoms of anaemia and debility, while left-sided lesions produce symptoms of advancing obstruction, that is, change of bowel habit and cramping abdominal pain, which may progress to frank obstruction. This difference occurs because the right colon is relatively wider and transmits a more liquid stool than the left colon (so that right-sided cancers can bleed and cause debility 'quietly'), while left-sided tumours tend to be the stricturing type, compared to the 'cauliflower' lesions which usually develop in the right colon.

363 The characteristic features of a rectal cancer are its shape, consistency and sometimes its fixity. It is usually possible to feel that the lesion is a raised, irregular ulcer, so that the finger rises over the rolled edge, and into the central depression. Cancer feels very firm, unlike the softer, benign lesions. If the cancer has penetrated the wall to involve extrarectal structures, there is a sensation of absolute or relative fixity compared to the mobility of normal tissue. Rectal cancers above ten centimetres from the anal verge are not usually palpable at all.

364 One should start from the premise that the patient has cancer until proven otherwise, though other conditions, such as polyps, villous adenomas, diverticular disease and inflammatory bowel disease, can also produce these symptoms. After careful physical examination including digitation of the anus and proctosigmoidoscopy, a barium enema is mandatory. If after clinical examination and radiology the diagnosis is not clear, colonoscopy should be performed.

365 Anterior resection for cancer involves removal of a segment of the rectum and sigmoid colon together with the lymphatic drainage, followed by anastomosis of the colon to the rectal remnant. Abdominoperineal excision, however, comprises the complete removal of the rectum and anus by a combined approach via the abdomen and the perineum, followed by the formation of a permanent colostomy. Anastomosis after anterior resection is usually achieved by a conventional suture technique, but recently, the development of a transanal stapling device has allowed anastomoses to be performed for low cancers previously only removable by abdominoperineal excision.

366   As with most radical operations for cancer, large bowel procedures comprise removal of the primary lesion together with its lymphatic drainage in the hope that this will achieve removal of all malignant tissue. As the nodes and lymphatics draining the colon and rectum lie along the arteries to the bowel, the relevant arteries are traced to their source, and flush-tied, followed by their removal with the involved segment of bowel.

367   This is a system of pathological staging applied to operative specimens, and has been shown to provide the most precise prognostic information available at the time of primary treatment. The Dukes' system describes a Stage A, in which there is spread of growth into the submucosa or muscle but not beyond, and with no lymph node involvement; Stage B, when the tumour penetrates through bowel wall without node involvement; and Stage C, in which, whatever the spread within or through the bowel wall, lymph nodes are involved. Over 90 per cent of Stage A patients can expect to survive at least five years, while for Stages B and C, the corresponding figures are about 60 per cent and 30 per cent respectively.

368   This is done as a safety precaution to allow the anastomosis to heal satisfactorily and thus prevent the serious consequences of anastomotic breakdown. This manoeuvre is used if the anastomosis has been technically difficult, and hence perhaps less sound than usual, or if the bowel has not been satisfactorily prepared mechanically before the operation. The colostomy is usually closed six to eight weeks after the main procedure, after checking the anastomosis by barium enema.

369   Ulcerative colitis, familial polyposis coli and simple adenomatous polyps. The risk of malignancy in ulcerative colitis is especially important in those with total colitis, and among those in whom the disease developed at a young age. If these two criteria are present, the risk of cancer having developed within 25 years of the onset of colitis is up to 40 per cent. In those with familial polyposis coli, in which the large bowel mucosa becomes covered by thousands of polyps, malignancy will always supervene if prophylactic colectomy is not performed. As far as simple adenomatous polyps are concerned, there is evidence that most carcinomas arise from these lesions, though most polyps do not progress to malignancy.

370   Although the theory is by no means proven, it is commonly believed that the initial problem lies in the low fibre content of the Western diet. This leads to low volume, firm stools, the passage of which is difficult,

leading to colonic muscular hypertrophy, greatly raised intraluminal pressure, and finally the forcing out of mucosal diverticula next to the blood vessels piercing the bowel wall along the edges of the taeniae coli.

371 Very. Although usually asymptomatic, it can be shown radiologically that one-third of the population have this condition at the age of 60, and two-thirds at 80.

372 Most commonly, diverticular disease presents with flatulence, a sensation of bloating and lower abdominal pain or discomfort. The bowel function is variable, but often with a tendency to pass small, pellet-like stools. If pain is present it is usually described as like 'wind pain', and may be mainly in the left iliac fossa. All these symptoms are presumed to be due to activity of the hypertrophic colonic muscle.

373 First, the nature of diverticular disease should be explained to him, indicating the need to increase the roughage content of the diet with the aims of eradicating present symptoms and preventing future complications. Then he should be given instructions regarding a high fibre diet, and asked to use this as part of his daily routine in future. The instructions include the use of unprocessed bran (mixed with the breakfast cereal) and wholemeal bread, and the regular intake of fruit and vegetables.

374 Acute diverticulitis; pericolic abscess; peritonitis, either faecal due to perforation of a diverticulum, or purulent due to rupture of a pericolic abscess; haemorrhage; fistula formation; and obstruction. All develop due to infection or erosion around diverticula. Infection occurs readily in the narrow-necked diverticula, leading on to a generalized inflammatory process (diverticulitis), which unusually may cause obstruction of the lumen of the bowel. Suppuration in an inflamed area leads to a pericolic abscess, which can rupture into the peritoneum, or into a nearby organ, particularly the bladder, producing a fistula. Finally, erosion at the neck of a diverticulum can lead to perforation, or haemorrhage from the blood vessel next to it.

375 The important diagnosis that may not have been excluded is colonic cancer, as the muscle hypertrophy induced by the diverticular disease can make the spotting of a malignant stricture difficult. If the surgeon or radiologist is unhappy, a colonoscopy should be performed as this is the only investigation that can properly exclude malignancy.

376 There are two types of rectal prolapse—incomplete, in which only the mucosa protrudes, and complete, in

which the whole thickness of the rectal wall prolapses, constituting an intussusception of the distal bowel through a weakened pelvic floor. Incomplete (mucosal) prolapse can occur at any age, while complete prolapse occurs mainly in young children and old ladies, especially those who have a long history of straining at stool.

377 Surgery offers the only possibility of cure in this age group. The commonest and most satisfactory procedure is the Ivalon rectopexy, in which, via an abdominal approach, the rectum is fully mobilized, a sheet of Ivalon sponge is placed into the sacral concavity and the rectum sutured to it; subsequent fibrosis prevents prolapse. Other procedures are less satisfactory— anterior resection is more risky, while the more minor Thiersch operation, in which a wire or nylon suture is placed around the anus, usually leads to faecal impaction, and often fails ultimately due to breakage of the suture.

378 The complications of ulcerative colitis can be divided into local and systemic. Local complications include toxic megacolon, perforation, massive haemorrhage, benign stricture and carcinoma. The first two require urgent surgery, while haemorrhage alone rarely leads to operation. Benign strictures develop in about 10 per cent of patients with chronic disease and must be differentiated from cancer. Malignant change occurs mainly in those with total colitis and a long history, and in whom the initial attack was severe. Systemic complications, most of which are uncommon or rare, include arthritis, especially ankylosing spondylitis; skin conditions such as erythema nodosum and pyoderma gangrenosum; eye lesions—iritis and episcleritis; and hepatobiliary problems such as cirrhosis, sclerosing cholangitis and bile duct carcinoma.

379 There are emergency, urgent and elective indications for surgery in ulcerative colitis. The emergency indications are the acute complications—perforation, toxic megacolon and continuing massive haemorrhage. Surgery is required urgently in the fulminating case not responding to several days of aggressive medical treatment, while elective surgery is required for carcinoma, severe dysplasia (indicating imminent malignant change), chronic debility or stunted growth in the pubertal patient. The usual elective procedure is proctocolectomy with ileostomy. In emergencies, or if the rectum is relatively mildly affected, the rectum may be left in situ, the proximal end being brought out as a mucous fistula; later an ileorectal anastomosis may be fashioned, or the rectum excised.

380 Crohn's disease affects the large bowel in about one-third of patients, either alone or in combination with small bowel disease. When Crohn's disease affects the large bowel it produces symptoms akin to ulcerative colitis, that is, diarrhoea and bleeding, often with weight loss and general debility. Very commonly it affects the anus, producing fissures which may be multiple, abscesses and complex fistulae.

381 By far the commonest cause of fresh bleeding per rectum is piles. However, major bleeding usually arises from colonic lesions, especially diverticular disease and angiodysplasia, which is a vascular malformation usually located in the right colon. The possibility of carcinoma must always be considered.

382 No—most patients settle on bed rest and blood transfusion. If haemorrhage continues or recurs, surgery must be considered; selective arteriography is the investigation of choice to locate the site of haemorrhage so that the appropriate bowel segment can be resected. Barium studies and endoscopy rarely locate the site of active haemorrhage and therefore are not usually employed in this situation.

383 Large bowel polyps may produce the same symptoms as cancer—bleeding and mucous discharge. Sometimes rectal polyps prolapse through the anus, and may be mistaken by the patient for piles. Frequently polyps are asymptomatic and multiple, so that detection of rectal polyps on sigmoidoscopy calls for examination of the rest of the bowel by double-contrast barium enema and colonoscopy.

384 Ninety five per cent of colonic polyps and all rectal polyps can be removed without recourse to abdominal surgery. Pedunculated colonic lesions and sessile polyps up to about 2.5 cm in diameter can be removed via the colonoscope using a diathermy snare. Bleeding becomes a significant possibility in the treatment of lesions over 2 cm, so these patients should be admitted and blood cross-matched prior to endoscopy. Rectal lesions, if solitary, can simply be removed via the rigid sigmoidoscope, or by submucous excision under general anaesthesia if large or wide-based.

The anus and anal canal

385 Puborectalis, the upper part of the external anal sphincter, is vital for faecal continence. The rest of the external sphincter and the internal sphincter can be divided, as, for example, in fistula surgery; such extensive division may produce incontinence of flatus

or of very loose stool, but normal stool can be controlled so long as puborectalis remains intact.

386   The lower half of the anal canal is lined by squamous epithelium, while the rest is lined by rectal-type mucosa. The distal part of the skin-covered area contains anal glands and has hair. The transition between the skin and mucosa occurs at the dentate line, which is often very tortuous, with islands of either cell type to be found above and below the line.

387   Piles arise in the vascular tissue deep in the mucosa in the upper anal canal, usually in the left lateral, right posterior and right anterior positions (otherwise known as 3, 7 and 11 o'clock positions). They sometimes expand deep to the mucosa to cross the dentate line so that skin covers their inferior poles. Additionally, a ring of so-called external pile tissue, often circumferential rather than three separate areas, may be found under the skin close to the anal verge.

388   The commonest symptom is bleeding on defaecation, usually first noted as blood on the toilet paper. Other symptoms include discomfort after defaecation, pruritis ani and prolapse which may or may not require manual reduction. Pain is unusual, except when piles become strangulated, or if another lesion, such as a fissure, is coexistent.

389   Many patients make a self diagnosis of piles if they pass blood. The doctor must never omit digital examination and proctosigmoidoscopy to exclude more serious causes of bleeding—this usually requires referral to hospital. Unless the symptoms and endoscopic findings all point towards piles as the cause of bleeding, and especially in the over 40s, it is best to perform a barium enema—change of bowel habit, passage of mucus, abdominal pain, weight loss, the finding of blood or free mucus in the rectum all demand this investigation. In short, piles are so common that a possible co-existing lesion higher in the bowel must always be energetically excluded if clinical findings suggest the need.

390   There are three degrees of piles—first-degree piles cause symptoms, usually bleeding, but do not prolapse; second-degree piles prolapse but reduce spontaneously; while third-degree piles prolapse and require manual reduction. First-degree piles are best treated by sclerosant injection, and correction of any constipation with a high fibre diet. Second-degree piles can be treated either by injection or by the use of the elastic banding technique, while third-degree piles can be banded if small enough, or removed by haemorrhoidec-

tomy if large, especially if there are accompanying skin tags. Today only five per cent of pile patients require haemorrhoidectomy.

391   I would remember that this is called reactionary haemorrhage, and that it may be due to minor ooze from the cut surface which should respond to conservative measures, but can also be a major bleed from a single vessel which will require further surgery to stop it. Having checked the vital signs and seen the extent of the external bleeding, I would elevate the foot of the bed, which may 'take the pressure off the piles', calm the patient, using sedation if necessary, take blood for cross-match and put up a drip if the bleed seems serious. I would alert my senior colleagues, who would decide to return to theatre if the haemorrhage were large or persistent.

392   An anal fissure is a longitudinal ulcer, usually in the posterior midline of the distal anal canal, and is often, though not exclusively, associated with constipation and sphincter spasm. The patient gives a history of variable length, most often complaining of pain and bleeding on defaecation, perhaps with pruritis or a discharge; the bleeding is usually only noticed on wiping. On examination a sentinel skin tag and the lower part of the fissure may be seen on gently parting the buttocks. Gentle digital examination may reveal sphincter spasm and induration around the fissure. If proctoscopy is not too painful to perform, it will demonstrate the length of the fissure, perhaps with the internal sphincter visible in its base, and a proximal fibrous anal polyp if present.

393   A fistula-in-ano is an abnormal communication between the anal canal (or rarely the lower rectum) and the perianal skin. It arises following an infection in one of the anal glands, which open into the anal canal at the dentate line and which ramify in the space between the internal and external sphincters. The infection may spread down this intersphincteric space or through the external sphincter into the ischiorectal fossa, either way then bursting through onto the perianal skin. Thus the majority of fistulae open internally at the dentate line (via the anal gland in which the infection started), while the site of the external opening is variable. Other ramifications are less common. The diagnosis is based on a history of continuous or intermittent perianal discharge, perhaps with occasional abscess formation, and the finding of an external opening on the perianal skin and an internal opening in the canal—the latter is sometimes only confirmed at operation.

394   Anal fistulae can only be treated surgically. At operation the first aim is to define the anatomy of the

lesion accurately using probes. Next the track is laid open by dividing all tissue superficial to it by cutting down onto a probe in the fistula; the wound is then lightly dressed. Treatment continues on the ward, with once or twice daily baths, irrigation, and light redressing of the cavity, aiming to induce healing in the deeper part of the wound first. The major danger of operation is that the surgeon may not recognize that a high fistula passes through or even above puborectalis—if he then divides all tissue superficial to the track, he would divide the sphincter, causing faecal incontinence.

395 Perianal abscess arises as an extension from infection in the intersphincteric space. Thus it is sited close to the anal verge, in the area between the lower borders of the internal and external sphincters. Ischiorectal abscess arises in the ischiorectal fossa, outside the whole sphincter mechanism, and bounded deeply by the levator ani, and laterally by the ischium; therefore it tends to point further away from the anus than a perianal abscess.

396 These abscesses should be drained via a skin incision sufficient to allow gentle digitation to break down loculi. The anatomy of the lesion should be confirmed, and an internal opening into the anal canal sought. However, if such an opening is found, division of muscle, as in fistula operation, should be deferred, as the anatomy may be very distorted by inflammation, causing confusion and perhaps iatrogenic incontinence—it is better to perform a further EUA at a later date to deal with such a track. After drainage the wound is lightly dressed daily until healing or the next EUA.

397 The most common disease causing perianal sepsis is Crohn's disease. Others include tuberculosis and leukaemia, the latter sometimes causing particularly extensive and troublesome lesions.

398 All types of anal malignancy are uncommon, but the lesions most frequently encountered are squamous cell carcinoma, arising at the anal verge, and basaloid carcinoma, which occurs in the lower anal canal. Adenocarcinoma can arise above the dentate line, while melanoma also usually arises high in the canal. While adenocarcinoma spreads to the abdominal nodes, like rectal cancer, the other tumours spread first to the lymph nodes in the groin.

399 As anal warts are usually sexually transmitted, all patients should be screened for other diseases. In particular the rectum should be checked for gonococcal

proctitis, and mucus sent for a culture if appropriate, and blood must be taken to screen for syphilis and hepatitis B.

400 This is the term applied to a localized area of thrombosis in the veins beneath the perianal skin; it is otherwise known as a thrombosed external haemorrhoid. It presents as a severely painful perianal lump, which may be small, spherical and blue, or rather more diffuse and lighter in colour. It is initially very tender, but this usually eases after several days.

The breast

401 Lymph from the breast drains medially and laterally. The medial half of the breast drains predominantly to the nodes situated along the internal mammary artery, which runs behind the anterior ends of the ribs; the lateral half of the breast drains to the axillary nodes, which lie along the medial axillary wall from the tail of the breast to the apex of the axilla.

402 The three major causes of nipple discharge in order of frequency are duct ectasia, intraduct papilloma and intraduct carcinoma. Typically, duct ectasia leads to a dirty green discharge from several orifices on the nipple, and may be bilateral on careful examination. Papilloma or carcinoma cause a discharge which may be bloody and can be localized to a single duct on the affected nipple.

403 The two symptoms may be unconnected. However, malignant pleural effusion occurs in 50 per cent of patients with breast carcinoma at some stage of the illness; the possibility that the lump is malignant and that the patient has a pleural effusion must be seriously considered.

404 A malignant breast lump may produce deformity of the affected breast, dimpling of the overlying skin, inversion of the nipple or peau d'orange; sometimes skin ulceration may be present. Breast cancers are very variable in size, so this factor does not aid differential diagnosis. The edges of a malignant breast lump are usually ill-defined, the surface irregular and the consistency very firm. With more advanced lesions fixity to skin and pectoral muscles may be detected.

405 Both of these physical signs strongly suggest that a breast lump is malignant. Tethering is due to malignant involvement of the fibrous bands (ligaments of Astley-Cooper) which connect the skin of the breast to the pectoral fascia; it produces dimpling or

decreased mobility of the skin overlying the lump, but some mobility is maintained. Fixity implies direct spread of the malignancy into the skin, preventing any 'sliding' of the skin over the lump by the examining hand. Fixity is a sign of locally advanced disease, while tethering, of itself, carries no prognostic significance.

406 This is a presentation of breast cancer sometimes seen in the elderly. The patient often has no idea of the length of the history, and may be totally unperturbed by the lesion. The cancer causes the breast to contract markedly so that sometimes no normal tissue remains. The scab represents an area of ulceration. Although these lesions are obviously locally advanced, there is frequently no evidence of spread beyond the chest wall. The majority of such cases respond well to oestrogens, oestrogen antagonists or local radiotherapy, preventing the development of distressing symptoms.

407 The recent development of unilateral nipple inversion must be regarded as due to the presence of breast cancer until proven otherwise. If, as is usual, a lump cannot be felt deep to a recently inverted nipple, further investigation including mammography is mandatory to locate the causative lesion. Long standing inversion, unilateral or bilateral, has no sinister significance.

408 This is a condition in which one nipple develops an appearance identical to eczema; it is due to the development of an intraduct carcinoma which may, or may not, be palpable. Histology reveals the presence of large vacuolated cells with small, dark nuclei in the epidermis. This condition must be differentiated from true, simple eczema which is always bilateral and has no malignant association. When Paget's disease of the nipple is diagnosed, carcinoma can be assumed, and managed accordingly.

409 This is a physical sign usually associated with breast cancer, but sometimes seen with a breast abscess. The skin overlying the lesion literally takes on the appearance of orange peel; it is due to lymphatic oedema caused by the underlying disease.

410 This is due to lymphoedema, which occurs when the axillary nodes become damaged or destroyed by the presence of secondary growth, by radiotherapy or by surgical removal in radical mastectomy. The arm becomes swollen, sometimes enormously, making it heavy and difficult to use. Rarely, it causes lymphosarcoma. Lymphoedema occurs in about 5 to 10

per cent of patients who have had radiotherapy or radical surgery.

411 A breast cancer should never be regarded as sufficiently 'clinically obvious' to exclude the need for histological confirmation. This can be obtained by taking tissue using a biopsy needle or by fine needle aspiration as an out-patient, or by excision under general anaesthetic with frozen section, immediately prior to mastectomy. Some surgeons perform bone and liver scans, as well as the usual chest x-ray and liver function tests, prior to surgery for breast cancer, especially if knowledge of the degree of occult spread will affect the extent of the operation.

412 Yes. Histological confirmation of cancer at the earliest stage in management takes much of the suspense out of the situation, allowing surgeon and patient to confront the diagnosis and plan management on a more positive basis.

413 Cytology is the study of isolated cells. Examination of cell morphology allows the pathologist to give the clinician some idea of the nature of the lesion, particularly whether it is malignant. Some surgeons use fine needle aspiration cytology in the diagnosis of breast cancer; it is perhaps less sensitive than needle biopsy, but if positive it facilitates rational management.

414 Radiology helps us to assess the primary lesion and to look for secondary spread. X-ray of the breast (mammography) is a high definition technique which discriminates between soft tissues of different densities; this allows detection of breast lumps, even if impalpable, and defines their outline, a help in differential diagnosis. Even better definition is produced by xeromammography. Distant spread is sought using chest x-ray, skeletal films, and bone and liver isotope scans as appropriate. Brain secondaries are best detected by CT scan.

415 The state of the axillary nodes is the single most important factor in assessing prognosis in breast cancer. Ten years after primary treatment, around two-thirds of patients whose axillary nodes were free of disease will still be alive, compared to one-third if there was nodal spread.

416 The commonest sites for distant spread are bone, liver, lungs and pleura, in that order.

417 For many years it was assumed that breast cancer spread in stepwise fashion, that is, that the primary enlarged, followed by lymph node involvement and

finally generalized, blood-borne dissemination. More recently it has been suggested that widespread occult micrometastasis may occur at an extremely early stage, and that the appearance, or not, of obvious dissemination reflects host response to the tumour. The first of these theories resulted in the concept that 'the more radical the operation, the greater the chance of cure'. However, radical local surgery has not affected the incidence of distant spread. This has lent support to the theory of early occult metastasis and has resulted in a more conservative surgical approach to the primary disease.

418 These terms have been in use for a long time attempting to separate those patients in whom treatment holds some prospect of cure—the 'early' cases—from those in whom cure is very unlikely, so that palliation should be the aim of management. In more precise terms, 'early' refers to patients with tumours which are T2 N1 M0 or less, using the TNM classification, that is, in whom the primary tumour is 5 cm or less in diameter, and disease outside the breast is limited to mobile axillary nodes on the same side as the primary lesion. The concept of 'early' and 'advanced' disease may be useful in practice, but holds connotations of stepwise spread which may be erroneous.

419 Halsted was Professor of Surgery at Johns Hopkins University, USA, at the end of the last century. He described the classical radical mastectomy in 1896, which some still use, and which is alleged to have produced the first cures of breast cancer.

420 Simple mastectomy is an operation in which the whole of one breast, and no other tissue, is removed. Radical mastectomy involves removal of a breast, together with its axillary lymphatic field. Complete node clearance requires removal of one or both of the pectoral muscles, to allow access to the apex of the axilla. In the 'classical' radical mastectomy the breast, nodes and both pectoral muscles are taken en bloc, while the 'modified' or 'Patey', radical procedure leaves the pectoralis major intact.

421 Surgeons and radiotherapists around the country differ widely in their attitudes to extent of surgery and the use of radiotherapy in the potentially curable case. However, on the basis of controlled trials, radiotherapy has been shown to have no effect on survival, but decreases the incidence of local recurrence, especially in patients who have undergone simple rather than radical mastectomy, and particularly if the axillary nodes are known to be involved. Many clinicians would

advocate a policy involving simple mastectomy and axillary node sampling, with radical radiotherapy if the nodes are involved; if the nodes are clear, radiotherapy can safely be deferred until the onset of local recurrence in the minority developing this complication.

422　The patient is usually fitted with an external prosthesis, though several surgical replacements are also possible. Normally the patient wears a light, temporary prosthesis in her bra for the first six weeks, and later can choose from a variety of devices, either of soft foam or filled with liquid silicone or glycerine to mimic the normal texture. In some circumstances, especially in the patient unable to accept the mutilation that has befallen her, a mammoplasty, to build an internal replacement of the breast, using a prosthesis or muscle or omental grafts, can be performed, but not usually within the first year or two after mastectomy.

423　There are four main patterns. First, some tumours become locally advanced, with no evidence of distant spread; typically this group is represented by the ulcerating scirrhous lesion in an old lady. Second, a patient may present with an apparently 'early' primary, but be found on investigation to have distant spread. Third, distant spread or local recurrence may develop after previous radical treatment of an 'early' primary tumour. Fourth, a patient may present with symptoms due to distant disease, such as bone pain, and be found on examination to have a small, previously unnoticed breast primary. Each of these situations will require a different management approach.

424　Two sorts of surgery can be considered in the treatment of advanced breast cancer—surgery to the primary, and various endocrine ablative procedures. Removal of the primary tumour, if not 'locally advanced', is usually performed in patients with distant spread to prevent distressing progression of disease on the chest wall; the usual operation would be simple mastectomy. Endocrine ablative procedures, oöphorectomy, hypophysectomy and adrenalectomy— which frequently produce remissions in advanced cases—have been largely superseded by medical ablative treatment.

425　Pain is the major mode of presentation for bone metastases—about half of all patients with distant spread in breast cancer require treatment for this problem. The other major mode of presentation is pathological fracture—the commonest sites are in the vertebral column, sometimes causing paraplegia, and in the femur. Pain from bone secondaries is usually rapidly relieved by irradiation. Early mobilization is important after fractures, as these patients have a short prognosis, so femoral fractures are best pinned and irradiated. Spinal lesions are sometimes an indication for laminectomy to try to alleviate or prevent spinal cord compression.

426   There are two forms of endocrine manipulation in advanced breast cancer—medical and surgical. Medical techniques include administration of oestrogens, tamoxifen (an oestrogen receptor antagonist), and the adrenal steroid synthesis inhibitor, aminoglutethimide. Surgical procedures comprise oöphorectomy, hypophysectomy and adrenalectomy. The first choice in premenopausal women is still probably oöphorectomy, while in the postmenopausal, oestrogen or tamoxifen therapy are first-line approaches. Major endocrine ablation has been superseded by aminoglutethimide, which should be reserved for use in relapse following successful first-line treatment. Remission occurs in about 30 per cent of patients in response to endocrine therapy, and more frequently if oestrogen receptors are present in the primary tumour.

427   Youth is no protection against breast cancer, though most cases do occur after the age of 35. Even the most 'benign feeling' lump, in an otherwise blameless breast should be removed at any age, as cancer can only be excluded histologically.

428   A breast mouse is a fibro-adenoma. This term was coined at some time in the past to characterize the mobility of this lesion—it seems to run away and hide when touched by the examining hand.

429   A cyst is usually ovoid, firm, fairly discrete and smooth; it is not as mobile as a fibro-adenoma. Unlike other cysts, lesions in the breast cannot be tested for fluctuance or transillumination as they are deeply placed. The most important confirmatory physical sign is successful, complete aspiration of fluid so that the lesion disappears.

430   Generalized lumpiness is usually due to fibro-adenosis. This condition occurs most commonly in multiparous women, especially towards the menopause. Usually a segment of the breast is involved, while sometimes the area is small, mimicking cancer by its vague outline and its irregularity. Fibro-adenosis is not dangerous and is best left alone, but any question of cancer in a small nodular area must be resolved by open biopsy.

431 The cardinal clinical feature is discharge from the nipple which is either bloody or brown. Palpation will often reveal a small lump deep to the areola, pressure upon which produces further discharge from the nipple, confined to the opening from the relevant duct.

432 Not very much. It cannot be assumed, even after mammography, that a breast lump is benign until it has been removed. However, lumps which subsequently prove benign on histology, particularly fibro-adenomata or cysts, have a characteristically smooth outline with no microcalcification on mammography, unlike the usual features of a cancer.

433 The residual lump should be removed. Although it is likely that it is due to benign fibrocystic disease, a carcinoma may be present, so excision biopsy is necessary to exclude this.

434 Careful questioning will usually reveal that the pain occurs around period time—such pain is thought to be related to the changes in hormone levels associated with menstruation, and is termed cyclical mastalgia. So long as no discrete lump is present, the woman should be reassured straight away that she does not have cancer. If persistent and severe, the pain may be relieved by danazol, a synthetic progestin, or by bromocriptine, which affects prolactin production, but both drugs may induce side effects.

435 There are two histological patterns in fibro-adenoma, the pericanalicular and the intracanalicular; both have a well-defined capsule, and both have an epithelial element in a fibrous tissue stroma. In the pericanalicular lesion, the epithelium forms ductules within the fibrous tissue, while the intracanalicular fibro-adenoma comprises fibrous tissue projecting into the duct system, which is thus stretched over it as a single layer of cells.

436 The best mimic of breast cancer is fat necrosis, which occurs after trauma to the breast. It presents as an irregular, ill-defined breast lump, sometimes with skin tethering; a history of trauma does not exclude cancer, as many women ascribe breast tumours to this cause. Excision biopsy is mandatory. Bloody nipple discharge, often thought to be a sign of intraduct carcinoma, is in fact usually due to benign papilloma; again, histology must be sought. Nipple inversion may suggest malignancy but if it is long standing, and especially if bilateral, it is innocent. Finally, nipple eczema can mimic Paget's disease of the nipple but is always bilateral.

437 Breast abscesses occur most commonly in breast feeding mothers, in whom the milk forms the perfect

culture medium. Occasionally neonates lactate under the influence of transplacental maternal prolactin, so they occasionally develop breast abscesses. Finally this lesion can occur in menopausal women in whom hormone fluctuations lead to secretions which can become infected.

438 A segment of the breast becomes painful and throbbing. On examination there is erythema, perhaps peau d'orange, induration and tenderness in the affected area. These signs are sufficient indication for surgery. Fluctuation is a late sign in breast abscess, and should not be awaited.

439 Sometimes—if a patient, probably a lactating mother, is seen within a few hours of the onset of localized pain, and there is tenderness and induration locally, then a course of an antibiotic such as flucloxacillin may prevent development of an abscess. Usually, however, patients are seen at least 24 hours after symptom onset, and in this group antibiotics will probably have no useful effect and may mask the symptoms and signs, allowing extensive abscess formation before proper surgical treatment is finally given.

440 As with all abscesses, a breast abscess needs adequate incision and drainage. This entails incision over the apparent centre of the lesion (fluctuation is not usually present to guide the surgeon), digital breakdown of loculi, despatch of pus for culture and light dressing of the cavity to prevent premature closure. Antibiotics and inhibition of lactation are not normally required.

441 The usual organism is *Staphylococcus*, which probably infects the breast by passage from the nasopharynx of the suckling infant.

442 This term literally means 'female breast' and refers to the condition in which breast tissue develops abnormally in the male. This happens frequently at puberty, usually resolving spontaneously; it can also develop in other situations in which hormone imbalance occurs, including cirrhosis (impaired clearance of hormones from the blood), stilboestrol therapy for prostatic cancer, and the abnormality of sex chromosomes, Klinefelter's syndrome. Treatment is only required in patients in whom it persists, causing embarrassment—subareolar excision of the breast disc is the procedure used.

443 The term mammoplasty covers both surgical enlargement and reduction in breast size. Enlargement can be performed in women whose natural breasts are very small—the usual technique is the submammary placement of an appropriately sized

plastic sac containing liquid silicone. A similar technique, or a procedure involving the incorporation of a pedicle graft of omentum or latissimus dorsi, can be used to replace a breast after mastectomy. Reduction mammoplasty, in which massive breasts are decreased to normal size, retaining the nipple, is indicated in young women who have abnormally large, pendulous breasts which have proven uncomfortable and unattractive.

The endocrine system

444 The thyroid develops from the median bud of the pharynx and descends from the base of the tongue to its position in the neck. Arrest of descent can occur at any point. A lingual thyroid is found at the base of the tongue and may be the only functioning thyroid tissue present. A median ectopic thyroid is found as a midline swelling in the upper part of the neck. A thyroglossal cyst can form anywhere along the line of normal thyroid descent. Sometimes the cyst can become infected and rupture, forming a so-called thyroglossal fistula.

445 Inorganic iodide is taken up by the gland, oxidized to iodine and bound to tyrosine to form either mono- or di-iodotyrosine which combine to form T3 (tri-iodothyronine) and T4 (thyroxine).

446 The serum levels of T3 and T4 are measured by radio-immunoassay. The T3 uptake test is a measure of the capacity of iodine binding sites and when used in combination with serum T4 levels gives a value for the free thyroxine index (FTI = T4/T3 uptake × 100). Thyroid stimulating hormone (TSH) can be measured by radio-immunoassay and is most useful in the diagnosis of hypothyroidism. Thyroid scanning with I^{131} or Technetium^{99} will reveal areas of functioning or non-functioning thyroid tissue.

447 This indicates an area of low or non-function, usually due to a cyst or a colloid nodule, but in about 12 per cent of cases it represents a neoplasm. A cold nodule should therefore be viewed with suspicion and explored surgically or, if cystic, perhaps aspirated under ultrasound control.

448 Non-toxic goitre is caused by an inadequate amount of iodine in the diet as may occur in mountainous areas where it is sometimes endemic. It can also be due to a congenital defect in the enzymes responsible for the uptake and utilization of iodide, or the presence of

substances in the diet capable of blocking the uptake of iodide, such as thiocyanate which is found in vegetables of the brassica family.

449 There are mixed areas of hyperplasia, involution, degeneration and normal tissue—it is thought that this pattern is due to a variable response to TSH in different parts of the gland. In hyperplastic areas the follicles are lined by columnar cells and contain colloid which is scolloped around the periphery, while in areas of involution the follicles may be enlarged or even cystic. Interspersed amongst these areas are fibrous scars and focuses of old haemorrhage.

450 Thyrotoxicosis may be due to a primary overactivity of the gland which becomes uniformly enlarged and vascular (Graves' disease), toxic transformation in a long-standing nodular goitre, or occasionally from a solitary autonomous adenoma in the gland. Rarely, overdose with thyroxine replacement may produce symptoms and signs of thyrotoxicosis.

451 The patient is anxious and irritable. There may be a history of weight loss, diarrhoea, polydypsia, and intolerance of hot weather. On examination, there is tachycardia, sometimes atrial fibrillation, exophthalmos, tremor and increased sweating; the thyroid is symmetrically enlarged and a bruit may be present due to increased vascularity. Besides exophthalmos eye signs include lid lag and, in more severe cases, defects in eye movement due to myopathy or conjunctival infection due to extreme proptosis.

452 Antithyroid drugs work either by preventing the uptake and concentration of iodide by the gland (for example, potassium perchlorate), or by inhibiting the oxidation of iodide and the binding of iodine to tyrosine (for example, carbimazole). Carbimazole is the most commonly used drug; once the patient has been rendered euthyroid a maintenance dose is continued for one to two years. Propranolol is used to counteract the cardiovascular effects of thyrotoxicosis and is particularly useful in the pre-operative preparation of a thyrotoxic patient.

453 Radioactive iodine is usually reserved for patients over the age of 40 because of the dangers of radiation to the gonads and to the thyroid glands of growing children and women of child bearing age. It is particularly useful for recurrent thyrotoxicosis. It is uniformly effective but there is a high incidence of eventual hypothyroidism.

454 Surgery is indicated when medical treatment fails to render the patient euthyroid; following relapse after

carbimazole therapy; when the patient does not comply with medication; or if sensitivity reactions to carbimazole, such as agranulocytosis, develop. Surgery is the treatment of choice in toxic nodular goitre as this responds poorly to medical treatment.

455 The patient is rendered euthyroid with carbimazole and propranolol. Lugol's iodine is given for a sennight pre-operatively to reduce the size and vascularity of the gland. The patient is admitted to hospital several days pre-operatively to check that she is euthyroid. Indirect laryngoscopy is performed to confirm normal pre-operative cord movement; serum calcium should also be checked. Two units of blood are cross-matched.

456 Most apparently solitary thyroid nodules are part of a nodular goitre, the remainder of which is not clinically detectable. A truly solitary nodule may be a cyst, a carcinoma or an adenoma—the latter may produce thyrotoxicosis. A thyroid scan will differentiate between functioning and non-functioning areas—so called hot and cold nodules; cold nodules should be viewed with suspicion and further investigated by ultrasound and aspiration cytology or exploration as 12 per cent of these are malignant.

457 Surgery is performed for nodular goitre to treat or prevent compression of the trachea and oesophagus by the goitre itself or haemorrhage into it; to remove the unsightly lump; or if the nodular goitre has become toxic.

458 The specific complications of thyroidectomy are haemorrhage, vocal cord paralysis, hypocalcaemia and thyroid crisis. Haemorrhage in this region is particularly dangerous as it can cause suffocation. One or both cords may be paralysed due to recurrent laryngeal nerve damage; this causes stridor and hoarseness. Hypocalcaemia follows accidental removal of the parathyroid glands and is manifested by tetany. Thyroid crisis, a very rare complication nowadays, is a very severe form of thyrotoxicosis, and only occurs if a toxic patient has been inadequately prepared pre-operatively.

459 Primary thyroid carcinomas may be papillary, follicular, anaplastic or occasionally medullary. Secondary tumours in the thyroid are very unusual.

460 This is in fact a metastasis from a papillary thyroid carcinoma which has replaced a cervical lymph node. As it is usually well differentiated it was previously thought to be ectopic normal thyroid tissue.

461 Papillary carcinoma usually occurs under the age of 40, is often multifocal and metastasizes to regional lymph nodes. Follicular carcinoma tends to occur in older patients and blood-borne spread to lungs and bone is common. The prognosis with either tumour is fairly good, but particularly with papillary lesions, so long as recurrent disease is detected early and treated.

462 Papillary tumours are usually multifocal, with early spread to regional nodes. The operation of choice is therefore total thyroidectomy and excision of involved nodes. As follicular carcinoma tends not to be multifocal, thyroid lobectomy may be adequate local treatment; however, total thyroidectomy has the advantage that it facilitates effective treatment of disseminated disease with radio-iodine postoperatively as this is then exclusively concentrated by metastatic tumour. In both cases full thyroid replacement is given to reduce the TSH stimulation of any residual tumour.

463 There are three eponymous types of thyroiditis—Hashimoto's, de Quervain's and Riedel's. Hashimoto's disease is auto-immune and presents as hypothyroidism; de Quervain's thyroiditis is probably due to a viral infection and presents with pain and fever; in the very rare Riedel's thyroiditis there is dense fibrosis of the gland which may cause tracheal compression and laryngeal nerve palsy and is sometimes associated with retroperitoneal fibrosis. Acute suppurative thyroiditis is very rare.

464 Hashimoto's thyroiditis usually occurs in 30 to 50 year old females. Initially the gland is enlarged, smooth and may be slightly tender and at this stage the patient may be hyperthyroid. As the condition progresses the patient becomes hypothyroid and eventually the gland becomes fibrotic and impalpable. The diagnosis is usually confirmed by finding antithyroid antibodies though sometimes biopsy is required to clinch it. Treatment is usually confined to thyroid replacement therapy, though sometimes surgery is required for cosmetic reasons or to relieve pressure.

465 There are usually four parathyroid glands arranged in pairs behind the upper and lower poles of the thyroid lobes. The upper pair develops from the fourth pharyngeal pouch, while the lower pair develops from the third pouch and migrates caudally with the thymus, sometimes ending up in a retrosternal position. Identification at operation can be difficult unless they are enlarged but they have a characteristic yellowish brown appearance. The glands selectively take up methylene blue and this can be given pre-operatively to aid identification.

466 Primary hyperparathyroidism is due to excess
production of parathormone, usually by one or more
parathyroid adenomata, though in about 10 per cent of
cases generalized parathyroid hyperplasia is the cause
and rarely carcinoma. Secondary hyperparathyroidism
may develop in chronic renal failure or intestinal
malabsorption, both of which interfere with the normal
dietary intake of calcium, leading to increased
parathyroid activity. In tertiary hyperparathyroidism
one or more glands, in a patient already suffering from
secondary hyperparathyroidism, becomes
adenomatous and continues to produce increased
amounts of parathormone.

467 Hyperparathyroidism may present due to the effects of
hypercalcaemia or to the symptoms caused by
abnormal bone metabolism. Hypercalcaemia most
commonly presents with nephrocalcinosis and renal
calculi, but can also cause abdominal pain, muscle
weakness and mental disturbance; in others peptic
ulceration or pancreatitis develop. A raised serum
calcium may be an incidental finding on biochemical
screening. Other patients present with bone disease
(osteitis fibrosa cystica, or Von Recklinghausen's
disease of bone) in which demineralization, the
formation of bone cysts and 'brown tumours'
(tumour-like masses of osteocytes) lead to pathological
fractures.

468 Elevated serum calcium levels should be confirmed on
several occasions and parathormone assayed. Typical
radiographic features occur in the hands—
subperiosteal bone resorption of the middle
phalanges, tufting of the terminal phalanges and cyst
formation. If on the basis of these investigations
primary hyperparathyroidism is likely, the neck is
explored to obtain confirmation of the diagnosis and to
treat it.

469 Regular checking of serum calcium may pick up
hypocalcaemia before it causes trouble. Hypocalcaemia
may provoke spontaneous carpopedal spasm, while in
others there will be Trousseau's sign (carpopedal
spasm on occluding the brachial artery with a blood
pressure cuff), Chvostek's sign (facial twitching on
percussion of the facial nerve) or mental disturbance.
Immediate treatment with calcium gluconate (10 ml
10 per cent solution) followed with calciferol and oral
calcium supplements is indicated.

470 Cushing's syndrome is caused by excessive circulating
glucocorticoids. The commonest cause is medical
treatment with steroids but spontaneous cases are
usually due to bilateral adrenal hyperplasia, which

may be secondary to a pituitary or bronchial ACTH-producing tumour. Adrenal adenoma or carcinoma are other possibilities.

471 The typical features are a moon face, greasy skin and acne, a fat trunk with thin limbs, hypertension, and impotence or amenorrhoea. Abdominal striae are usually present and there may be marked osteoporosis. Diabetes is common.

472 Conn's syndrome is due to excess aldosterone production from the adrenal cortex, usually due to an adenoma. This produces sodium retention and potassium depletion leading to muscle weakness, cramps, polyuria, headaches and hypertension.

473 Adrenalectomy is the treatment of choice in patients with Cushing's or Conn's syndrome where hyperplasia or an adenoma of the adrenal cortex is the cause. This operation is now rarely used in the palliation of advanced breast cancer.

474 Aminoglutethimide, which inhibits steroid synthesis (especially oestrogens) by the adrenal cortex and other tissues can be used to induce 'medical adrenalectomy', particularly in advanced breast carcinoma.

The arteries, veins and lymphatics

475 The two main symptoms are intermittent claudication and rest pain. Claudication strictly means limping, but by general usage the term intermittent claudication refers to a severe cramp-like pain, usually in the calf, precipitated by exercise and relieved by rest, and indicates an inadequate blood supply to exercising muscles. Rest pain is felt in the toes and feet, is usually worse at night and relieved by hanging the foot out of bed. It implies there is severe peripheral ischaemia even under resting conditions, and gangrene and amputation are inevitable unless arterial reconstruction can be performed.

476 About 70 to 80 per cent of claudicants are unchanged or improved over a five-year period and only 20 per cent require surgery, with 10 per cent needing amputation. In diabetics the risk is higher with 20 to 30 per cent requiring amputation. There is, however, a 20 per cent mortality in claudicants up to 12 years from the onset of claudication, mainly from myocardial infarction.

477 During sleep the blood pressure, pulse rate and cardiac output all fall, reducing peripheral perfusion below a

critical level, producing pain which wakes the patient, who will often hang his leg out of bed to seek relief.

478   The major established risk factors are systemic hypertension, obesity, cigarette smoking, diabetes, and hyperlipoproteinaemia. Epidemiological studies have established a direct relationship between systolic blood pressure and atherosclerosis; reduction in blood pressure reduces the incidence of atherosclerosis-related complications. Obesity promotes the development of hypertension. Smoking in excess of 20 cigarettes per day is also an established risk factor, cessation of smoking reducing the risk particularly following myocardial infarction. Diabetes and Frederickson's types II and III hyperlipoproteinaemias are associated with the development of premature atherosclerotic disease.

479   The three areas most prone to atherosclerosis are in the arterial supply of the lower limb—the aorto-iliac segment, the femoral bifurcation and the superficial femoral artery, and the popliteal trifurcation and below. Aorto-iliac disease produces thigh and buttock claudication which, when associated with absent femoral pulses and impotence, constitutes Leriche's syndrome. Femoral disease produces calf claudication and the effects may be more severe than aorto-iliac disease as the limb is often totally dependent on femoral blood flow with little collateral supply at this level. Distal disease, that is atheromatous disease distal to the popliteal artery involving the small vessels of the popliteal trifurcation and beyond, is not usually amenable to surgical reconstruction.

480   The commonest conditions to be confused with intermittent claudication are sciatica and osteo-arthritis of the hip or knee. Sciatica often has a similar pain distribution to intermittent claudication and the associated paraesthesia in the foot can simulate rest pain. The pain of osteo-arthritis is often aggravated by exercise. Less commonly, a condition known as intermittent claudication of the cauda equina, due to bony narrowing of the spinal canal, produces pain and neurological signs on exercise.

481   Examination of the cardiovascular system should include assessment of the pulse and blood pressure, palpation of the carotid arteries and listening for bruits. Abdominal examination is important to look for an aneurysm. The lower legs and feet should be examined for their nutritional state, muscle wasting, pallor, cyanosis, and areas of ischaemia and gangrene. The nails often lose their normal sheen and trophic ulcers may be apparent over bony pressure points such

as the metatarsal heads. Pallor and venous guttering may be provoked by elevation, and cyanosis by hanging the leg down (Buerger's test). The temperature of the skin of the legs at various levels should be compared by simple palpation. Femoral, popliteal, posterior tibial and dorsalis pedis pulses should all be palpated and the presence of femoral bruits ascertained.

482 Femoral bruits are caused by turbulent flow in the femoral vessels and indicate significant atheromatous narrowing in the aorto-iliac segment.

483 The patient should be told to stop smoking, lose weight if necessary, avoid temperature extremes, take particular care of his feet to minimize trauma and the risk of infection, and to commence a programme of regular exercise which may improve the claudication distance. Finally, the patient should be reassured that his symptoms are likely to remain static or even improve if he adheres to this advice.

484 Claudication distance should be objectively measured on a treadmill. Ankle systolic pressures can be measured using a pressure cuff and a Doppler probe. In normals the ankle pressure is unchanged or increased slightly after exercise but falls in obstructive arterial disease—the time to return to pre-exercise values is related to the adequacy of the collateral supply. More sophisticated investigations include ultrasound analysis of the pulse wave form at various points in the arterial tree, and a pulsatility index and transit time can be calculated. Arterial flow can be measured by occlusion plethysmography, isotope clearance and electromagnetic flow measurement.

485 This is the ratio of the ankle systolic pressure to the brachial systolic pressure. Normally this is greater than 1.0. Claudicants usually have values less than 0.8, and values of less than 0.5 are associated with rest pain and indicate severe ischaemia.

486 Aortograms should be reserved for patients in whom surgery is being contemplated, that is, patients with severe rest pain, gangrene, deteriorating claudication distance or in whom claudication is severely limiting their daily activities. The aim of the investigation is to define the anatomy of the disease so as to determine the feasibility of surgery and the choice of procedure.

487 A translumbar aortogram (TLA) usually requires a general anaesthetic and involves a direct puncture of the abdominal aorta below the level of the renal arteries. A transfemoral aortogram using the

Seldinger technique, in which a catheter is inserted over a guide wire via the femoral artery into the aorta, is performed under local anaesthetic but can be difficult if there is marked atheromatous disease in the femoral vessels. Complications include subintimal dissection, extravasation of contrast, and haematoma formation in the retroperitoneum or in the groin with the risk of subsequent formation of a false aneurysm.

488 Atherosclerosis is a disease of the large elastic and muscular arteries. The earliest identifiable lesion is the fatty streak caused by subintimal lipid deposition. This progresses to the typical atheromatous plaque composed of cholesterol, phospholipids and triglycerides covered with a layer of collagen, while the internal elastic lamina becomes fragmented. The plaques are liable to ulceration and thrombosis on their exposed surfaces or haemorrhage into them. These processes may lead to stenosis or to weakening of the vessel wall causing aneurysm formation.

489 It is not clear whether atherosclerosis is primarily a disease of the vessels, the blood constituents or a combination of both. Cholesterol and phospholipids can cross the endothelial surface and excess lipid deposition occurs as a result of either a local increase in endothelial permeability or a decrease in the mechanisms which normally clear plasma-derived molecules from the vessel wall. Smooth muscle proliferation occurs in response to subendothelial injury and platelet adherence. The precise mechanisms which control these processes are unknown.

490 General advice regarding exercise, obesity and smoking should be given. Co-existing medical conditions such as anaemia, polycythaemia, hypertension and diabetes all require treatment. There is little evidence to suggest that vasodilator drugs or those which alter blood viscosity are of any value. Acute ischaemia may be helped by infusions of dextran or prostacyclin in some cases.

491 Sympathectomy can be performed either surgically or chemically. A surgical sympathectomy consists of excising the L2–L4 lumbar sympathetic ganglia and the intervening sympathetic chain via an extraperitoneal approach. It is usually performed in patients unfit for major reconstructive surgery or in whom such procedures are technically impossible. A chemical sympathectomy is performed by direct phenol injection. The effect of sympathectomy is dilatation of skin vessels without improving muscle blood flow. Therefore it is useful in relieving rest pain

and in promoting healing of ulcers but is of no value in the treatment of claudication. The benefit is temporary.

492   Atherosclerosis is commoner, occurs at a younger age and is more rapidly progressive in diabetics. In addition the small vessels are often involved. Neuropathy causes painful paraethesiae or loss of pain and temperature sensation. Motor neuropathy leads to small muscle atrophy and the development of clawed toes, which in turn leads to soft tissue damage by the shoe. Infection is difficult to eradicate because of impaired blood supply. There may also be abnormal arteriovenous shunting contributing to tissue hypoxia and increased platelet activation.

493   The most likely causes of an acutely ischaemic leg are emboli (from the heart, from aneurysm, or from an atheromatous plaque) and acute thrombosis on pre-existing leg vessel atheroma. Less common causes are trauma from a fracture or penetrating wound, an aortic dissection and vasospasm due to frostbite or ergot poisoning.

494   The patient's own long saphenous vein or a variety of foreign materials can be used for arterial reconstruction. Autogenous saphenous vein is the best material for reconstruction below the inguinal ligament and for coronary artery surgery but its use is limited by its size and availability. Teflon or Dacron grafts never completely endothelialize and so are thrombogenic, particularly at low flow rates, and are therefore mostly used in aorto-iliac surgery. Recent alternatives to saphenous vein are the glutaraldehyde-treated umbilical vein and Goretex grafts, both of which are non-thrombogenic.

495   In descending order of magnitude the operations available are replacement with a bifurcation graft, which these days has a low operative mortality and good long-term patency rates; local endarterectomy; axillobifemoral grafts, used in patients unlikely to withstand major abdominal surgery; and percutaneous balloon angioplasty for localized stenoses.

496   This term refers to grafts which shunt blood, ignoring normal anatomy, to overcome ischaemia in patients in whom major aortic reconstruction is impossible, or contra-indicated due to intercurrent disease or local sepsis. The commonest are the axillofemoral and the femoro- femoral cross-over grafts; both are tunnelled subcutaneously. The axillofemoral graft is used in cases of bilateral aorto-iliac disease, whereas a

femorofemoral graft can only be used if a single iliac vessel is occluded.

497 The commonest sites for atheroma to develop are at its origin from the bifurcation of the common femoral artery and where it leaves the adductor canal through the hiatus in adductor magnus.

498 When the superficial femoral artery becomes occluded the lower leg relies on the profunda femoris for its blood supply. Often the origin of the profunda itself is narrowed but it rarely becomes totally occluded. Profundaplasty (in which an endarterectomy and patch insertion are used to enlarge the lumen of the proximal profunda) is used as a limb salvage procedure or as part of a more major vascular reconstruction such as aortofemoral graft.

499 A clinically significant reduction in flow is apparent only when there is a 70 to 80 per cent stenosis although experimental work on pulsatile flow shows that much less marked stenosis has a measurable effect on flow dynamics.

500 The usual procedure is a femoropopliteal bypass graft from the common femoral artery to the popliteal artery below the occlusion, or on occasion to the posterior tibial or peroneal artery if the popliteal is occluded. The best graft material is autogenous saphenous vein which is removed and reversed so that valves do not obstruct arterial flow. If this is unavailable or of poor quality then one of the newer graft materials such as Dardik biograft (glutaraldehyde treated umbilical vein) or Goretex (polytetrafluoroethylene) should be used.

501 The important factors are graft material, distal run-off and smoking. Reconstructive surgery above the inguinal ligament with a Dacron graft has a patency of 75 to 80 per cent at five years. Below the inguinal ligament where the flow is less, the five-year patency is less than 50 per cent in spite of the use of saphenous vein.

502 The indications are gangrene, ulceration, persistent infection, and severe incapacitating rest pain in a limb in which revascularization is impossible. As a general principle the knee joint should be preserved to produce a better functional result; this can only be done if clinical ischaemia is confined to the distal lower leg and foot. Further, surgery should be more radical in the very sick patient who cannot withstand later revision, while it can be much more conservative in diabetics.

503　An aneurysm is an abnormal dilatation of an artery, usually due to atherosclerotic weakening of the arterial wall; these aneurysms can be fusiform, when the vessel is circumferentially dilated, or saccular, when there is an asymmetrical 'blow out'. Aneurysms can also be caused by infection (mycotic aneurysm), trauma, and connective tissue diseases (e.g., Marfan's syndrome). The term is used loosely in the conditions known as false aneurysm and dissecting aneurysm.

504　A false aneurysm is a lesion in which the wall of the sac is formed not by the true constituents of the arterial wall but by organized fibrous tissue and haematoma, although the sac does communicate with the arterial lumen. It results from a contained arterial leak which may be due to penetrating trauma (knife wound, fracture, arteriography), blunt trauma, pathological rupture, or at the site of vascular anastomosis.

505　An aortic dissection is the result of a spontaneous tear in the aortic intima and inner part of the media, usually due to atheroma and hypertension. Blood then tracks between the inner and outer layers of the media forming a double-barrelled aorta. Untreated, rupture into the thorax, pericardium or abdomen usually occurs with a fatal result although occasionally spontaneous rupture back into the aortic lumen more distally decompresses the dissection.

506　An aortic dissection presents with severe pain in the chest, back or abdomen, which may mimic other conditions such as myocardial infarction or perforated peptic ulcer. As the dissection proceeds the branches of the aorta may become progressively occluded causing ischaemia of the brain, spinal cord, gut, kidneys and lower limbs with the appropriate clinical syndromes.

507　Surgery is the treatment of choice in dissections involving the ascending aorta whereas those confined to the descending aorta are best managed conservatively, with controlled hypotension. The reason for the more aggressive approach in the ascending group is the likelihood of death from aortic valve failure, coronary artery occlusion or rupture into the pericardium if surgery is not carried out. On the other hand, surgery of the descending thoracic aorta carries a serious risk of spinal cord ischaemia and should therefore be avoided if possible; surgery may be required, however, if there is progressive widening of the aorta, indicating incipient rupture.

508　Abdominal aneurysms may be found incidentally on examination or when calcification of the wall is seen on x-ray. As they enlarge they may become symptomatic causing abdominal discomfort or more frequently, back pain due to erosion of vertebral bodies. Pressure on surrounding organs may produce symptoms such as vena caval compression or ureteric obstruction. Rupture is often preceded by increasing pain but sudden rupture presents as an acute abdominal catastrophe or sudden death. Occasionally the aneurysm is found following massive bleeding into the gastro-intestinal tract, or following embolism into the legs.

509   The extent and size of the aneurysm should be determined with plain x-rays, particularly the lateral view, looking for calcification, and more accurately by ultrasound or CT scanning, to define the upper limit in relation to the renal arteries. Surgery is indicated in most cases, unless the aneurysm is small or the patient is unfit to withstand major surgery. At operation, the aorta is controlled above and below the aneurysm, the sac opened and a Dacron tube graft inserted. If the aneurysm extends to involve the iliac arteries, then a bifurcated graft is used.

510   Approximately 60 to 70 per cent of aneurysms rupture within two years of being noticed and although the operative mortality of symptomless aneurysms is in the region of 10 per cent this rises to 75 per cent once they have ruptured. Thus if the patient is otherwise fit, surgery should be advised particularly if the aneurysm is more than 7 cm in diameter.

511   No, some aneurysms are not resectable. The minority of aneurysms that extend above the renal arteries are not usually regarded as suitable for surgery as replacement of thoracic and abdominal aorta is a formidable undertaking. Inflammatory aneurysms, which are uncommon, provoke a marked reaction in the retroperitoneal tissues, so that surgery would be extremely hazardous. Various less radical procedures may be considered which include filling the aneurysm with coils of stainless steel wire or wrapping it with an external support such as Marlex mesh.

512   Iliac, common femoral, popliteal, subclavian, axillary, brachial and carotid arteries may all be sites of aneurysm formation. Occasionally multiple sites will be involved and this may have a familial incidence. A generalized dilatation of vessels with aneurysm formation at some sites may occur as a variation of atherosclerosis and is called arteriomegaly. John Hunter was the first surgeon to describe a treatment for peripheral aneurysms when, 200 years ago, he performed proximal ligation for popliteal aneurysm.

513 An embolus is a body, foreign to the blood stream, which is transported from one part of the vascular system to another. Pulmonary embolism is the commonest type, originating from thrombus formed in the veins of the lower limb. Also fairly common is arterial embolism from thrombus formed in the fibrillating left atrium or the recently infarcted left ventricle; less common cardiac sources are prosthetic valves and atrial myxoma. Arterial emboli can also arise from the material deposited within aneurysms and from platelet aggregations formed on atheromatous lesions in the carotids. Air embolus may enter the circulation via one of the large veins in the neck during surgery, fat embolism is a common sequel of major orthopaedic trauma, and tumour emboli may occur due to direct venous invasion, usually from renal tumours. Recently, therapeutic embolization using gelfoam or dura mater has been used to infarct tumours.

514 Emboli tend to lodge at arterial bifurcations, most frequently at the division of the common femoral artery. The effects depend on the size of the occluded vessel, the extent of the thrombosis which occurs secondary to the occlusion and, finally, the adequacy of the collateral circulation. Embolism to the leg presents with pain, coldness and pallor followed by sensory and motor deficit. If ischaemia is prolonged beyond eight hours the leg may be lost. Embolism to the brain presents with stroke, to the retina with blindness, to the kidney with pain and haematuria, and to the mesenteric circulation with a sometimes confusing history of non-specific abdominal pain, with rapid general deterioration.

515 Heparin, as a bolus injection of 10 000 units, should be given immediately to limit the extent of secondary thrombosis. The operation is usually performed under local anaesthesia. The common femoral artery and its branches are exposed through a vertical groin incision and controlled proximally and distally. The common femoral is opened and a Fogarty balloon catheter passed proximally and distally until free prograde and retrograde flow are obtained. Postoperative anticoagulation reduces the risk of thrombosis.

516 Arteries may suffer sharp or blunt trauma which may be accidental, malicious or iatrogenic. Penetrating wounds may partially or completely transect arteries. The soft tissue injury associated with a limb fracture may produce an intimal tear which with its associated thrombosis may occlude the artery. Damage to contiguous arteries and veins may produce an arteriovenous fistula. Leakage of blood at the site of an

arterial injury with subsequent organization leads to the development of a false aneurysm. Accidental intra-arterial injection sometimes occurs, most commonly during the induction of anaesthesia with thiopentone.

517 Buerger's disease, or thrombo-angiitis obliterans, is a condition of unknown aetiology which typically affects heavy smoking, young men aged 20 to 40. There is a progressive inflammatory process which causes damage to neurovascular bundles in the periphery of the limbs leading to gangrene of the fingers and toes. Treatment is far from successful and involves stopping smoking, sympathectomy and local amputations.

518 The surgeon will have been asked to perform a temporal artery biopsy. Temporal, or giant cell, arteritis may be complicated by the sudden onset of blindness, so if the diagnosis is suspected it should be confirmed by temporal artery biopsy and steroids started immediately.

519 This is a syndrome in which the digital vessels, usually in the upper limb, go into spasm causing pallor, followed by a painful reactive hyperaemia in which the fingers become red and swollen, and subsequently blue. Occasionally symptoms are so severe as to produce ulceration or gangrene. This phenomenon is usually secondary to another condition affecting the arteries of the limb.

520 A variety of conditions have been found to produce Raynaud's phenomenon. These include atheroma in the main vessels of the arm, Buerger's disease, cervical rib, connective tissue disorders, trauma, ergot poisoning and occasionally as a result of working with vibrating tools.

521 Raynaud's disease is said to be present if the phenomenon occurs without a demonstrable underlying cause; this is most commonly seen in young women. Abnormalities of blood viscosity, plasma fibrinogen, immunoglobulins and digital artery patency have been detected in some cases. Treatment is initially aimed at protection of the affected part from cold; some patients require vasodilator drugs or sympathectomy. Recently, plasmapheresis has been found to relieve symptoms.

522 The classical mode of presentation of carotid atheroma is the transient ischaemic attack (TIA) which occurs as a result of platelet embolism from the ulcerated atheromatous plaque. A TIA may last from minutes to hours and is followed by a complete recovery, so the diagnosis is usually made on the history. Dysphasia,

focal weakness, or focal sensory disturbance are characteristic, and visual disturbances, which range from blurring of vision to monocular blindness (amaurosis fugax), occur in about 20 to 30 per cent of patients. Carotid atheroma as the underlying cause is strongly suggested by the detection of a carotid bruit. In about 30 per cent of patients a completed stroke follows one or more TIAs, usually within three years. Sometimes a carotid bruit may be an incidental finding during a routine examination.

523 Five years after detection of the bruit only 30 per cent of patients will remain asymptomatic. Around 25 per cent will have suffered transient ischaemic attacks (TIAs) and about 15 per cent will have sustained a stroke; the remainder will have died from other causes (mainly related to other atherosclerotic disease).

524 Several new non-invasive techniques are available to assess the functional effect of carotid atheroma, including measurement of carotid to supra-orbital pulse transit time and ocular plethysmography. The anatomy of the lesion can be demonstrated by ultrasound, and if surgery is indicated arch aortography with selective catheterization of the carotid and vertebral arteries is performed.

525 Antiplatelet agents such as sulphinpyrazone and dipyridamole (Persantin), used alone, are probably ineffective in reducing the risk of stroke following TIA. Aspirin may reduce the risk of major complications but the magnitude of this reduction is uncertain. Anticoagulants are of no value unless the source of emboli is the heart.

526 Carotid endarterectomy is the standard operation. The carotid bifurcation is explored through a vertical neck incision. If after cross-clamping of the common carotid and external carotid arteries there is a significant fall in the internal carotid arterial pressure then a temporary intra-operative shunt is used to by-pass the area whilst the endarterectomy is performed. In patients undergoing carotid surgery for unilateral TIAs the operative mortality is usually less than 1 per cent and the incidence of post operative stroke less than 2 per cent. Recurrent TIAs in the opposite hemisphere usually occur in a further 5 to 10 per cent. Carotid surgery should not be performed shortly after a stroke because of the risk of haemorrhage into an infarcted area.

527 This is a condition in which exercise of the arm produces symptoms of dizziness, vertigo, giddiness and occasional blackout. It is caused by an occlusion or

stenosis of the subclavian artery so that exercise of the arm provokes reversed flow down the vertebral vessels. A bruit is usually present in the root of the neck and the radial pulse on the affected side is weak or absent.

528 Acute mesenteric ischaemia, which usually results from an embolus lodging in the superior mesenteric artery, presents with increasing abdominal pain and with early development of shock. A recent myocardial infarct or the presence of atrial fibrillation may point to the diagnosis. The physical signs may be relatively undramatic in the early stages, but typically include generalized tenderness, mild guarding and absent bowel sounds. Unfortunately, the small bowel and proximal colon are often dead by the time a laparotomy is performed.

529 The barium enema shows the characteristic 'thumb-printing' appearance due to mucosal swelling in the affected segment. Sometimes this appearance can be seen on the plain x-ray if there is air in the lumen.

530 This is a rare condition characterized by postprandial pain ('abdominal angina'), weight loss and steatorrhoea, and is due to stenosis of the origins of the coeliac and mesenteric arteries.

531 A glomus tumour is a small, red, raised lesion usually occurring in the fingers, often in the nail beds. The patient may complain of pain disproportionate to the size of the lesion and on examination it is exquisitely tender to localized pressure with the point of a pencil. The lesion consists of a small knot of arterioles and venules surrounded by nerve endings.

532 A carotid body tumour, or chemodectoma, arises from chemoreceptor tissue between the internal and external carotid arteries and presents as a lump in the neck in middle age. These tumours are often slow growing but they may be malignant, the vagus and hypoglossal nerves may become involved, and metastases occur in 20 per cent.

533 Aetiological suggestions include failure to adapt to an upright posture, congenital weakness of the venous valves or vein wall, prolonged standing, pregnancy and a low residue diet. Extensive ileofemoral thrombosis causing venous obstruction, and venous hypertension secondary to an arteriovenous fistula are rarer causes.

534 The patient is first examined lying down while skin pigmentation and ulceration are looked for. She is then examined standing (so that the veins fill) in order to record the extent and course of the varicosities arising

from the long and short saphenous systems. The patient should then be asked to cough—a thrill in the groin indicates saphenofemoral incompetence. To determine the precise level of other incompetent communications between the deep and superficial systems, the patient is asked to lie down and a tourniquet is applied to the leg after the veins have been emptied by elevation. Any rapid filling of the superficial system below the tourniquet, after the patient has stood up, must then be via incompetent perforating veins. If surgery is contemplated it is important to check the patency of the deep veins. This is done by exercising the leg with the tourniquet in place; if the deep system is patent the superficial veins become less prominent as they decompress into the deep system (Perthe's test).

535 Injection sclerotherapy is adequate treatment for below knee perforator incompetence, but surgery is required if there is incompetence of the saphenofemoral or saphenopopliteal junctions. Injection is the easiest and cheapest method and avoids admission to hospital. The sclerosant is injected into the incompetent perforators and a compression bandage is applied for six weeks while they thrombose; during this period the patient must walk several miles a day to prevent extension of thrombosis into the deep veins. Surgery, on the other hand, involves several days admission to hospital, tying and stripping of the appropriate veins, but only two weeks of bandaging. Although the early results of sclerotherapy are good there is a recurrence rate of between 65 and 90 per cent after six years. Recurrence following surgery is about 15 to 20 per cent at six years.

536 The oedema, induration, fibrosis and pigmentation are all consequences of deep vein thrombosis, leading to venous hypertension in the leg. The normal venous pressure in the superficial veins when standing is approximately 90 mmHg, equivalent to the column of blood from the heart to the ankle. During exercise the calf muscle pump empties blood from the deep veins and reduces this pressure. However, after deep vein thrombosis the venous valves are destroyed, particularly in the perforating vessels, and retrograde flow occurs into the superficial system, with a rise in pressure. This in time may lead to oedema, induration, fibrosis and ulceration. Pigmentation is due to haemosiderin deposition following leakage of red cells into the tissues, causing irritation and eczema.

537 The superficial veins are dilated, may pulsate and contain blood of a high oxygen saturation. A hum can be heard and there may be a collapsing pulse.

If the shunt is large, high output cardiac failure may occur. Congenital A–V fistula in a limb may cause overgrowth.

538 This is a developmental abnormality of lymphatics and consists of a mass of lymphatic cysts. It is usually found in the neck, jaw or axilla and is brilliantly transilluminable.

Burns

539 This is a convenient method of burn area assessment in which the body surface is divided into eleven areas, each of which constitutes about 9 per cent of the body surface; these areas are the head, each arm, the back and front of each leg, and the front and back of the trunk, each divided into top and bottom halves. In other words, the head and arms are 9 per cent each, the legs 18 per cent each, and the trunk 36 per cent. The remaining 1 per cent is conventionally ascribed to the male genitalia.

540 The rate of fluid loss from the burned surface is directly proportional to the area burnt, so that assessment of the area involved is vital in working out fluid replacement. Depth of burn must be determined as those areas where the burn is full thickness will require skin grafting. Deep burns also lead to destruction of red blood cells, so that assessment of depth and area combined help determine the need for blood transfusion.

541 Capillaries in the deeper layers of skin and subcutaneous tissue that have not been completely destroyed become widely dilated and of greatly increased permeability; this leads to a disturbance in normal fluid exchange, resulting in loss of circulating volume as exudate from the raw surface, and as oedema.

542 This requires careful fluid replacement. If the burn is not too severe this can be achieved via the oral route, but in the more serious case intravenous replacement will be required. By about 48 hours post burn the excessive fluid loss ceases, so that fluid replacement (as opposed to normal maintenance) is necessary only during the acute phase.

543 There are three basic causes. First, during the acute phase dehydration and reflex renal vasoconstriction to compensate this can lead to acute renal failure. Second, in extensive deep burns, the release of tissue

breakdown products and haemoglobin can cause acute
tubular necrosis. Third, in the patient who has
developed major infection, septicaemia can lead to
renal failure.

544 Fifteen per cent of total body surface in adults, and 10
per cent in children, who cope with burn shock less
well than adults. With burns less than this size, extra
oral fluids are usually enough to cope with the
pathological fluid loss.

545 The badly burned patient is usually very frightened, in
pain and in mortal danger. Immediate attempts should
be made to reassure and calm him, and treat his pain
with strong analgesia. At the same time all clothes
should be removed to allow assessment of the area of
the burn, so that fluid replacement can be planned. A
good IV line should be inserted, preferably by cut down
into an arm vein. In burns over 25 per cent a urinary
catheter should be inserted to help monitor fluid
balance. Sepsis should be pre-empted by early dressing
with antibacterial creams, such as Flamazine, or with
clean sheets as a first aid measure. Anyone with a burn
of more than 10 per cent should be started on a five-day
course of penicillin.

546 The first step is to estimate the burn area using the
rule of nines. Next it is important to remember that
the rate of fluid loss, and hence replacement, is highest
in the first 12 hours, thereafter decreasing until it
stops, usually at about 36 hours. A useful formula can
be used to plan fluid replacement based on this
changing rate of loss; the formula is based on the
'ration' of fluid, one ration being given four-hourly for
the first 12 hours post burn, six-hourly in the next 12,
and one ration in the third 12 hours. The ration for a
particular patient is worked out by multiplying the
percentage area of the burn by the patient's weight in
kilograms, divided by 2, and expressed as millilitres of
fluid. This replacement fluid is usually given as
plasma. The patient must be carefully monitored, and
changes in the rate of infusion made if necessary. It is
important to remember that the usual daily
maintenance requirement of fluid, around 2 or 3 litres
of water and electrolytes, must be given in addition to
the replacement rations.

547 This depends on the area of full thickness burn, as this
degree of injury involves destruction of blood cells at
the time of the burn. Attempts must be made to decide
what proportion of a burn is full thickness; if more
than 10 per cent of the body has full thickness damage,
blood transfusion is indicated, roughly at the rate of
one unit per 10 per cent body area deeply burned. This

formula applies to adults—special formulae are required to decide on the right volume for children.

548 The appearance is usually helpful. Erythema or the presence of blisters suggest superficial damage, while brown or black leathery skin, or translucent skin through which thrombosed vessels are visible, are signs of full thickness damage. There is a group in between which is more difficult to assess—in these the pinprick test is useful. A sterile pin or needle is driven firmly through the skin into the subcutaneous fat. Pain indicates survival of nerve endings and hence of viable skin cells, while the absence of pain suggests, though does not prove, that a burn is full thickness. There can, of course, be areas of full and partial thickness damage in the same patient.

549 Regular clinical assessment is vital to allow adjustment of the fluid replacement as required. This entails observing the patient's colour, degree of restlessness, blood pressure and pulse, hourly urine output, haematocrit, and, if progress is unsatisfactory, central venous pressure.

550 Grafts are required in the treatment of full thickness burns. They can help decrease fluid loss and perhaps prevent infection if applied in the acute phase, while in the longer term, they produce a much more satisfactory scar than would occur if the wound were left to epithelialize from the surviving skin around the burnt area.

551 It is normal to wait 14 to 21 days for the slough to separate and for healthy granulation to cover the recipient site. In some cases, however, early excision of the burn will provide a clean site to receive the graft. A partial thickness graft is taken from an unburned area, preferably from the thighs or lower legs, but the arms or trunk can be used if necessary; the instrument usually used is the Humby dermatome. The skin is spread, raw surface upwards, on tulle gras and then cut into suitable strips to apply to the recipient areas. If very large areas are to be grafted, the skin can be made to go further by making multiple slits in it; the graft can then be stretched, producing a 'string net' appearance. In circumstances in which the area to be grafted is so large that the patient cannot provide enough autograft, cadaver or animal skin may be used.

552 Uncontrolled shock due to massive fluid loss, and uncontrolled septicaemia.

553 First, a major burn patient should be nursed in a clean, dry atmosphere in a side room, away from the normal activity of the ward. Staff treating the patient should

wear gowns and masks when entering the room, and a 'no touch' technique used. The burn itself can be treated either by the 'open' or 'closed' methods. The time-honoured open method involves allowing a hard crust to form on the burn, which effectively acts as a barrier to the entry of infection. Alternatively, the burn can be dressed or, more commonly today, covered liberally and frequently with a cream antiseptic such as silver sulphadiazine. This method is certainly more useful in patients with more than one surface burned, or if the burn crosses a joint surface, movement of which would crack the traditional crust.

554 *Staphylococcus pyogenes* and *Pseudomonas aeruginosa* are the most important organisms. *Pseudomonas* produce much pus which will destroy surviving skin and float off grafts—it can also lead to septicaemia. Bowel organisms also appear frequently, spreading to the burn from the anal region.

555 It may kill immediately by its cardiac effect. The area where the lightning struck will have an irregular branched area of burn which will usually be full thickness. The current passing through the patient to ground may produce burning of muscle without damage to surface skin along the way, except at the site of exit, usually the feet. Bones may be fractured due to violent muscle contractions.

556 There are few definite rules. Patients with large areas involved benefit particularly from the sterile environment provided in special units. Those with full thickness burns to the face or hands, or with full thickness burns of any part adding up to more than, say, five per cent should ideally be transferred so that expert repairs can be performed. Other patients' site of management will depend on the interest in burns of the referring surgeon and on the availability in the area of a burns centre. Special units will always help with telephone advice, even if they do not take the patient.

557 Those who have been exposed directly to much flame or hot smoke may suffer burns to the air passages; this is a very serious, potentially lethal injury. Any patient at risk of having sustained such an injury must be monitored very carefully, both clinically and with blood gases. Antibiotics and vigorous physiotherapy should be used to try to prevent the development of pneumonia, and tracheostomy performed if respiratory function begins to deteriorate.

Paediatric surgery

558   Yes. The highest incidence of incarceration with subsequent risk of strangulation, and also damage to testicular blood supply, occurs within the first year.

559   The child is sedated and placed in gallows traction in which the feet are suspended by adhesive strapping from an overhead bar, with the bottom just off the mattress. In most cases spontaneous reduction occurs within an hour and a herniotomy should then be performed at the next elective list. The indications for urgent exploration are erythema of the overlying skin or other signs of strangulation, or failure to reduce on conservative measures.

560   Umbilical hernia occurs through a weak umbilical scar, usually as a result of infection. This type of hernia resolves spontaneously in more than 90 per cent of cases; if it persists, with no signs of getting smaller, it should be repaired around the age of three.

561   The surgical causes of neonatal breathing difficulties are tracheo-oesophageal fistula and congenital diaphragmatic hernia. TOF should be suspected if respiratory difficulties occur during feeding. When abdominal organs herniate through the diaphragm it is usually via the foramen of Bochdalek (persistence of the pleuroperitoneal canal).

562   There is often a history of maternal hydramnios. The baby may salivate excessively, and coughs and becomes cyanosed during feeds. Attempts to pass a fine catheter down the oesophagus will usually meet with failure. X-rays after 1 ml of lipiodol is introduced down the tube will confirm the diagnosis. If gas is present in the stomach then the distal pouch must be in communication with the trachea.

563   The usual presenting symptoms are regurgitation of all feeds and failure to thrive. If oesophagitis develops, bleeding or stenosis may ensue.

564   Conservative treatment is nearly always successful; the baby is kept upright continuously, antacids are given and the feeds thickened. Antibiotics and chest physiotherapy may be necessary. As the baby grows, the cardia descends into the abdomen. Oesophagitis is an absolute indication for surgery as complications develop rapidly—fundoplication is the procedure of choice. If a stricture develops a colonic interposition may be required.

565 Duodenal or small bowel atresia account for about 40 per cent of cases (about a third of babies with duodenal atresia have Down's syndrome). Hirschsprung's disease is the diagnosis in a further 25 to 30 per cent while meconium ileus, mid-gut malrotation and volvulus account for 15 per cent. Annular pancreas and internal hernia are rare causes. Neonatal intestinal obstruction occurs in about 1.25 per thousand births.

566 Repeated bile stained vomiting in the neonate is never normal and is almost invariably due to intestinal obstruction. However, if there is obstruction proximal to the ampulla, for example due to pyloric stenosis, the vomit will not contain bile.

567 Meconium is a thick viscid mixture of bile, digestive enzymes and shed intestinal cells. It has normally been passed by 18 hours after birth and delay in its passage may indicate intestinal obstruction. An inspissated plug of meconium may suddenly pass after a rectal examination.

568 Imperforate anus is one of the commoner congenital anomalies and might otherwise be overlooked in the first few days. Its severity can vary between an anal stenosis, in which there is no more than a membrane between the anus and the hind-gut, to more severe forms in which there is a large gap, often with a fistula between the rectum and urethra or bladder.

569 It occurs most frequently in first born males and there is often a family history. Regurgitation after feeds progresses to projectile vomiting between the age of two and six weeks. On examination, there is usually dehydration, evidence of weight loss, visible peristalsis, and a 'pyloric tumour' can usually be palpated during a feed.

570 Ramstedt's operation, or pyloromyotomy, is performed for this condition. It consists of splitting the hypertrophied pyloric muscle until the mucosa is free to bulge out. Pre-operative rehydration is important. Vomiting may continue for 24 to 48 hours post operatively.

571 Hirschsprung's disease presents either as neonatal intestinal obstruction or, later in childhood, as intractable constipation and failure to thrive; it is characterized by an absence of the myenteric plexus which involves the rectum and a variable length of colon proximal to it. Plain films show colonic distension and a barium enema shows a cone appearance where the dilated colon narrows into the distal aganglionic segment. In neonatal cases, a colostomy is performed to relieve the obstruction and a

full thickness rectal biopsy is taken to confirm the absence of ganglia. Later the aganglionic segment is excised and a pull-through operation performed to restore bowel continuity.

572 If barium enema reveals the typical 'coiled spring' appearance, if the intussusception has been present for less than 24 hours, and if there is no reason to suspect strangulation, then an attempt can be made to reduce the intussusception by the hydrostatic pressure of the column of barium. Usually, however, a laparotomy is required; the intussusception is manually reduced and bowel resected if necessary.

573 The most common causes are anal fissure and juvenile polyp. Fissure is caused by passing a hard stool and usually responds well to aperients and local lubricants. The juvenile polyp is a hamartoma, is usually single and is easily treated by diathermy snaring.

574 Chest and abdominal x-rays will reveal the position of the pin and whether it is open or closed. If the pin has lodged in the oesophagus, endoscopy is necessary to remove it, but if it has entered the stomach and is closed then treatment should be expectant—the parents should watch the stools for the pin and return if symptoms develop. If the pin is open, there is a risk of perforation; if still in the stomach it should be removed endoscopically, while if it has passed beyond the pylorus laparotomy may be required.

575 These are congenital urethral abnormalities. Hypospadias is the commonest congenital defect and occurs in 1 in 350 births. The external urethral orifice is situated on the under surface of the penis or scrotum. In addition the prepuce is hooded and the penis has a ventral curvature due to fibrosis of the corpus spongiosum. Surgical treatment consists of straightening the penis by freeing the fibrotic corpora and a new urethra created using skin flaps from the penis. Epispadias is much rarer—the urethra opens on the dorsal surface of the glans or penile shaft. If severe it may be associated with ectopia vesicae.

576 A hydrocele is a collection of fluid within the tunica vaginalis and in infancy it is due to a persisting processus vaginalis. It may disappear overnight after the child has been sleeping. Spontaneous resolution occurs if the processus closes but if it persists it is easily treated by surgical ligation of the processus.

577 Neonatal jaundice is common and usually physiological. The most likely surgical causes are biliary atresia, in which there is a progressive fibrous

obliteration of the extrahepatic bile ducts, and choledochal cyst; both lesions are rare.

578 This tumour, the commonest of childhood, is a haemangioma. It usually increases in size in the first year of life and can be unsightly but regression nearly always occurs so that treatment is rarely needed.

579 The commonest malignant tumours in childhood are neuroblastoma (which arises from the adrenal medulla or sympathetic ganglia), nephroblastoma (otherwise known as Wilms' tumour), and medulloblastoma.

580 Great improvements in treatment have occurred in the last two decades such that 60 to 80 per cent of children survive for two years. Nephrectomy is followed by radiotherapy and chemotherapy. In stage 1 (tumour confined to the kidney) and stage 2 (beyond the kidney but completely resected) radiotherapy is given to the renal bed followed by vincristine and actinomycin D for a year. In more advanced disease total abdominal radiotherapy is followed by intensive chemotherapy. Survivals of 85 per cent in Stage 1, 73 per cent in Stage 2 and 35 per cent in Stage 3 can be achieved.

The genito-urinary system

General points

581 Renal pain due to pyelonephritis, hydronephrosis or a tumour can vary from a dull, poorly localized ache in the loin to a severe throbbing pain with associated renal tenderness. Ureteric colic produces a remittent excruciating pain which typically radiates from the loin to the groin and often into the testis. Cystitis is usually accompanied by a suprapubic ache and scalding on micturition. Strangury is a particularly severe form of pain felt along the urethra and associated with an urgent desire to micturate and is often caused by a bladder stone. Pain in the prostate from prostatitis is usually poorly localized and felt in the rectum or perineum.

582 There are many lesions throughout the urinary tract that can cause haematuria but the commonest by far is acute cystitis. Tumours, stones, trauma, infections and other inflammatory conditions can affect any part of the urinary system and cause bleeding. In addition haematuria may be due to a generalized bleeding tendency such as thrombocytopenia or anticoagulant overdose. Less common specific conditions which may

present with haematuria are polycystic kidneys, renal infarction, Bilharzia and tuberculosis.

583 Initial haematuria, that is at the onset of micturition, usually originates from lesions in the urethra. Terminal haematuria is usually caused by abnormalities at the bladder neck or in the prostate. Total haematuria occurring throughout the stream gives little indication of the site of origin.

584 This should always arouse suspicion of an underlying renal anomaly such as hydronephrosis, tumour or polycystic kidney.

585 Lower urinary tract function is dependent on an intact autonomic and somatic nerve supply. Thus, occasional patients with neurological disease, such as multiple sclerosis, will present with urological symptoms, such as retention of urine, so lower limb and abdominal reflexes and assessment of anal sphincter tone should be performed in all patients.

586 100 000 organisms/ml of midstream urine indicates urinary tract infection. Infection should be suspected but is not proven by the presence of protein or blood on routine ward testing.

587 Sterile pyuria is a term used to indicate the presence of significant numbers of leukocytes in the urine in the absence of organisms on routine culture. Sterile pyuria, particularly in an acid urine, is highly suggestive of urinary tract tuberculosis. Other causes are bladder tumours, stones, and treated infection.

588 Providing renal function is normal, fluids are restricted for several hours prior to the investigation. A control film is taken looking for urinary tract calcification. An IV injection of contrast is given and films are taken immediately and at 5, 10 and 25 minutes with tomograms of the kidneys; compression may be applied to the abdomen to enhance filling of the renal pelvis. Later films may be required if there is delayed excretion. When the bladder has been adequately filled, an after micturition film is taken to assess bladder emptying. The immediate films will demonstrate the position, size and shape of the kidneys and by 5 minutes contrast will have filled the collecting systems and renal pelvis. The later films show position, size and architecture of the ureters and bladder.

589 These can be broadly classified into metabolic and non-metabolic. Stones may result from hypercalciuria, either idiopathic or secondary to hypercalcaemia as a result of hyperparathyroidism or Vitamin D overdose.

Less commonly, excess urinary excretion of uric acid, oxalates or cystine will cause stones. Non-metabolic causes include infection, immobilization, and persistently concentrated urine.

590 About 70 per cent of stones are formed from calcium phosphate or calcium oxalate in various proportions. Calcium oxalate stones occur either as small smooth stones, irregular mulberry stones or sharp spiky jack stones. Phosphate stones are usually a combination of calcium phosphate and magnesium ammonium phosphate often forming the large staghorn calculi which develop in alkaline, infected urine. Uric acid and cystine stones account for less than 10 per cent of the total and are usually hard and yellow.

591 Renal failure may be acute or chronic. Acute renal failure, indicated by sudden onset of oliguria, often progressing to anuria, may be due to prerenal, renal or postrenal causes. Prerenal causes include severe, prolonged hypotension or hypovolaemia due to burns, haemorrhage, septic shock or vomiting; obstruction to both kidneys is a postrenal cause. Chronic renal failure is progressive deterioration in function due either to intrinsic renal disease such as glomerulonephritis, or to prolonged obstruction.

592 There may be a history of long-standing prostatism or previous pelvic malignancy. Examination may reveal an enlarged prostate, a palpable bladder or a pelvic mass. A renal ultrasound is the most useful investigation as it will reveal evidence of hydronephrosis whereas an intravenous urogram is of limited value if the urea is markedly raised. There may be a rapid improvement in renal function following urethral or ureteric catheterization.

593 Pneumaturia is the passage of 'wind in the water'. This is virtually diagnostic of a vesicocolic fistula, due to either colonic diverticular disease or large bowel malignancy.

The kidney and ureter

594 On initial palpation the enlarged kidney is usually smooth while a notch may be felt on the inferior border of the spleen. On inspiration the spleen moves down, but the kidney may not. A renal mass can be made more obvious on abdominal palpation by pressure in the loin. Finally, on percussion the spleen is dull, while the kidney may seem resonant due to overlying bowel.

595 Blood urea is measured routinely but is not elevated until there is a 50 per cent reduction in renal function.

More sensitive measures of renal clearance and concentration include serum creatinine, creatinine clearance, urinary specific gravity and maximum urinary concentrating ability after fluid restriction. Individual renal function can be assessed using gamma camera renography.

596 The kidney can be abnormal in its structure, position or blood supply. The commonest abnormality is partial or complete division of the kidney and its collecting system into two moieties. The lower poles of the kidneys may be fused to form a 'horseshoe kidney'. Polycystic disease is another congenital abnormality. Rarely, one kidney may be absent. If a kidney is abnormal in position it is usually located in the pelvis. The commonest vascular abnormality is an aberrant lower pole artery arising directly from the aorta.

597 Tomograms help to delineate the lesion. An ultrasound examination will determine whether the mass is cystic or solid; a cystic lesion should then be aspirated by percutaneous puncture. Angiography is indicated if aspiration fails, reveals bloodstained fluid or if ultrasound suggests that the lesion is solid.

598 It is important for two reasons: to demonstrate a functioning, intact kidney on the uninjured side, and to obtain information about the injured kidney. An IVU may reveal unilateral non-function, suggesting major damage to the blood supply or varying degrees of discontinuity or extravasation.

599 Surgery is indicated for continued bleeding, the development of a mass in the loin, or secondary infection. At most, 25 per cent of patients with renal trauma require surgery and the aim of treatment is to preserve as much functioning renal tissue as possible.

600 Acute pyelonephritis presents with loin pain, fever and rigors, sometimes associated with dysuria, frequency and haematuria. The main physical finding is extreme loin tenderness. Infection is usually ascending rather than blood-borne and in over 50 per cent of patients is associated with an obstructive lesion of the urinary tract. The urothelium of the renal pelvis becomes inflamed and haemorrhagic and there is progressive parenchymal involvement sometimes with the formation of abscesses in or around the kidney.

601 The commonest organisms are *E. coli, Klebsiella, Proteus, Strep. faecalis, Micrococci* and *Pseudomonas aeruginosa. E. coli* accounts for 85 per cent of all cases, whilst the proportion due to *Proteus* and *Pseudomonas* is higher in hospital patients with surgical diseases,

having repeated instrumentations or on ineffective antibiotics.

602 The typical radiographic appearances of chronic pyelonephritis are shrunken kidneys, with calyceal clubbing and irregular cortical scars. The condition usually results from damage sustained in early childhood due to a combination of infection and vesico-ureteric reflux. In some patients progressive renal impairment occurs though continued infection is not always present.

603 Pyonephrosis is an abscess within the kidney, originating in the pelvicalyceal system, whereas a perinephric abscess is outside the renal capsule. Pyonephrosis results from acute obstruction to the ureter or pelvi-ureteric junction, with subsequent infection in the distended pelvicalyceal system, leading to rapid destruction of renal parenchyma. A perinephric abscess usually arises from an abscess within the renal cortex and only rarely as a result of septicaemia.

604 A small focus in the renal cortex, from blood-borne infection, may spread along the tubules to the medulla leading to ulceration at the apex of the pyramid, and in some cases to tuberculous pyonephrosis. The ureter becomes thickened, ulcerated and stenosed particularly at the lower end. A pyonephrosis may calcify—so-called autonephrectomy.

605 Three early morning urine specimens are examined for acid-fast bacilli on Ziehl-Nielsen stain and Löwenstein-Jensen culture. Plain x-ray may show renal calcification and an IVU may reveal irregular ulceration with destruction of calyces, evidence of ureteric fibrosis and contraction of the bladder. Anti-tuberculous drugs should be continued for about 12 months. Steroids may be given if there is evidence of ureteric obstruction as this may worsen, with loss of renal function. Surgery is rarely necessary.

606 The common causes of renal papillary necrosis are diabetes, analgesic abuse and sickle-cell disease. A papilla sometimes sloughs into the pelvis leading to an attack of ureteric colic.

607 Uric acid and cystine stones are radiolucent and account for less than 10 per cent of all urinary tract calculi.

608 Primary malignant renal tumours are of three main types—renal cell carcinoma, tumours of the pelvis and nephroblastoma. Renal cell carcinoma (hypernephroma) is the commonest renal tumour and

arises from the tubules. Tumours of the pelvis arise from the urothelium and are usually papillary transitional cell tumours but occasionally may be squamous if metaplasia has taken place as a result of infection or calculi. Nephroblastoma (Wilms' tumour) is a mixed tumour of epithelial and connective tissue arising from nephrogenic tissue, and is one of the commoner malignant tumours of childhood. Benign tumours, such as lipomas or fibromas, are rare.

609 Hypernephroma (literally meaning 'above-kidney-tumour') was originally thought to arise from adrenal tissue as it consists of large clear cells resembling those of the adrenal gland. This tumour is more accurately called a renal cell carcinoma today.

610 A persistent, low-grade pyrexia, often with anorexia and weight loss, occurs in 20 per cent, sometimes before any other manifestation of the tumour. Refractory hypochromic anaemia occurs in 30 to 40 per cent. Polycythaemia, hypertension and hypercalcaemia occur uncommonly, probably due to circulating polypeptides produced by the tumour. High alkaline phosphatase may occur in the absence of liver or bone metastases.

611 Renal cell carcinoma is treated by radical nephrectomy, through a thoraco-abdominal incision if necessary, excising the perinephric fat as well as the kidney. Postoperative radiotherapy may be given if there is evidence of spread beyond the renal capsule or if local nodes are involved. Pre-operative embolization is sometimes used to reduce vascularity or occasionally as an alternative to surgery. Transitional cell carcinoma of the renal pelvis is treated by nephro-ureterectomy as the whole urothelium is assumed to be potentially malignant. Regular follow-up is required to check the bladder, and the kidney and ureter on the other side.

612 ABO blood group compatibility between donor and recipient is essential as accelerated rejection occurs with incompatible grafts. The role of the HLA antigens is less well defined. The chance of finding a pair of siblings with the same four HLA antigens in common is 1 in 4; in kidneys transplanted between siblings, one year graft survival is significantly better in HLA identical grafts (90 per cent) compared to non-identical grafts (70 per cent). The results of parent-to-child grafting are similar to those in non-identical siblings.

613 Live related donors with good HLA match are the ideal, producing about an 80 per cent one year graft survival compared to 50 per cent for kidneys from

unrelated cadavers. Kidneys removed from cadavers often require preservation for several hours whilst the recipient is prepared, so that some are non-viable at the time of transplantation.

614 The most commonly used regime to prevent rejection is a combination of corticosteroids and azathioprine, with higher doses of steroids to treat episodes of rejection. Continuous steroid administration produces many problems so alternatives are being assessed; cyclosporin A either alone or with low doses of steroids is producing encouraging results. Antilymphocyte globulin and plasmapheresis are advocated by some but their use is controversial.

615 Part or all of the collecting system (renal pelvis and ureter) may be duplicated forming a duplex system. In complete duplication there are separate collecting systems draining the upper and lower poles of the kidney, with their ureters entering the bladder separately. The ureter draining the upper part of the kidney always enters the bladder lower than that draining the lower pole, and may end at an ectopic site such as the bladder neck or urethra. In lesser degrees of this abnormality, the renal pelvis is duplicated together with a varying proportion of the ureter, the separate systems joining to produce one ureteric opening into the bladder.

616 Bilateral hydronephrosis is usually due to conditions obstructing the lower urinary tract such as urethral stricture, benign prostatic enlargement, and carcinoma of the prostate or bladder. Advanced carcinoma of cervix or uterine body may involve both ureters. Bilateral ureteric obstruction occurs in retroperitoneal fibrosis and rarely with abdominal aortic aneurysms.

617 The patient complains of episodes of severe loin pain, often provoked by a diuresis. An intravenous urogram should be performed following the intake of a large volume of fluid; typically this will show a grossly distended renal pelvis with a normal ureter. Renography will confirm obstruction. Surgical treatment consists of a pyeloplasty in which the pelvi-ureteric junction is reconstructed either by resection and re-anastomosis (Anderson-Hynes operation) or by rotating a flap of the excess tissue of the renal pelvis to widen the narrowed segment (Culp's operation).

618 Urine should be tested for blood and an emergency IVU performed to confirm the diagnosis. The patient is given pethidine and an antispasmodic. In most cases

the calculus will be passed in the urine, which should be sieved in order to recover it, for analysis. Progress of the calculus may be followed with plain x-rays. Screening tests for underlying metabolic abnormality include serum calcium (to exclude hyperparathyroidism), 24-hour urinary calcium (to identify idiopathic hypercalciuria) and urinary cystine and uric acid.

619   Indications for surgery are complete obstruction; obstruction involving both or a single functioning kidney; the presence of infection; a stone judged too large to pass; repeated attacks of pain without progress of the stone; growth of the calculus; and association with an anatomical abnormality, such as a pelvi-ureteric junction obstruction.

620   This is a condition in which dense fibrosis occurs in the retroperitoneum, usually at the pelvic brim, encasing the ureters and obstructing them. The aetiology is unknown although methysergide, used in the treatment of migraine has been implicated; occasionally a malignant variety occurs in which retroperitoneal lymphatics become permeated with carcinoma from prostate, pancreas or breast.

621   The commonest cause is iatrogenic trauma during pelvic surgery. The upper ureter is occasionally injured by hyperextension injuries to the spine. The lower end of the ureter can be damaged by diathermy within the bladder or during Dormia basket extraction of a ureteric calculus.

622   Vesico-ureteral reflux is retrograde flow of urine from the bladder into the ureter during micturition. Reflux is relatively common in infants, but diminishes with age as growth of the bladder base tends to improve the competence of the mechanism at the vesico-ureteric junction. The diagnosis is made on a micturating cysto-urethrogram.

623   The aims of treatment are the prevention of recurrent infection; the reduction of reflux; and the minimizing of renal damage. Infections are treated promptly with appropriate antibiotics and long-term, low dose prophylactic antibiotics are used to prevent recurrent infections. Effective bladder emptying should be accomplished by practising double or triple micturition. The degree of reflux is assessed by micturating cystography, and progress monitored with three-monthly urine cultures, yearly urograms and renograms. Indications for ureteric reimplantation are failure to prevent recurrent infection; gross reflux; and progressive renal damage.

The bladder, prostate and urethra

624 There are several factors which cause urinary frequency in bladder outflow obstruction. The functional bladder capacity is reduced by the presence of residual urine and the encroaching middle lobe of the prostate; the hypertrophied detrusor becomes irritable and contracts inappropriately during bladder filling; and urinary infection stimulates the trigone.

625 The commonest cause is acute bacterial infection. In women this can occur without any obvious predisposing factor, while in men it is often a sequel to bladder outflow obstruction, its complications and treatment with a catheter. Sexually active women often complain of the symptoms of cystitis without demonstrable infection. Chronic cystitis may be due to tuberculosis, schistosomiasis or radiotherapy.

626 The final appearance is of a contracted fibrosed bladder with wide open 'golf hole' ureteric orifices. Initially tubercles form in the submucosa, particularly near to the ureteric orifices. These may eventually coalesce and ulcerate with subsequent fibrosis leading to a contracted bladder.

627 *Schistosoma haematobium*, which is the causative organism in Bilharzia, passes in the blood stream to the vesical venous plexus and sets up an intense inflammatory reaction leading to granuloma formation, ulceration and ultimately squamous carcinoma.

628 Exposure to the aromatic amines, benzidine, beta and alpha naphthylamine, has been found to increase the risk of developing bladder cancer thirty-fold. These substances are used in the chemical, rubber and cable industries; rat catchers used to use alpha naphthylurea in their poisons.

629 The usual presenting symptom is painless haematuria. Later frequency, dysuria and strangury develop, and if the ureters become obstructed the patient may develop renal failure. Presentation due to spread outside the bladder is uncommon.

630 Transitional cell carcinoma accounts for 95 per cent of cases. Squamous cell lesions may develop in areas of squamous metaplasia caused by stones or chronic infection, or within a diverticulum. Adenocarcinoma, associated with urachal remnants or ectopia vesicae, is rare.

631 All patients with painless haematuria should be investigated with an IVU, cystoscopy, and biopsy if

appropriate. Urine cytology may be a useful screening test in groups at risk. Tumours are staged by depth of invasion:

Tis—in situ carcinoma,
T1—papillary tumour not extending beyond lamina propria,
T2—invasion of superficial muscle,
T3—invasion of deep muscle or perivesical tissues,
T4—invasion of adjoining organs.

Staging is based on the cystoscopic appearance and careful bimanual examination under anaesthesia. Biopsies must include muscle wall to allow the pathologist to assess the degree of invasion. More recently, ultrasound and CT scanning have helped in staging.

632 Depending on the extent of the lesion, bladder cancer may be treated by transurethral resection (TUR), radiotherapy, chemotherapy or cystectomy. Superficial papillary tumours, 80 per cent of the total, are dealt with by TUR, followed by regular check cystoscopy. About half recur, and are treated with diathermy or TUR; superficial recurrence beyond endoscopic control may be treated with intravesical chemotherapy. Tumours extending deeply into muscle or beyond are managed with various combinations of radical radiotherapy, chemotherapy, and partial or total cystectomy, depending on the extent of invasion.

633 An ileal conduit is an artificial bladder, made from a segment of ileum which has been isolated with its blood supply. The ureters are implanted at one end and a spout ileostomy fashioned at the other. The indications for this procedure are total cystectomy for malignancy, or to bypass a severely malfunctioning bladder as may occur in spina bifida, and other neurological problems.

634 Bladder diverticula usually result from the increased pressure due to outflow obstruction, and follow compensatory detrusor hypertrophy, trabeculation and sacculation. They cause incomplete bladder emptying, stasis, infection, calculus formation and sometimes squamous carcinoma after metaplasia has occurred.

635 Urinary incontinence is an involuntary act of micturition which occurs when the intravesical pressure exceeds urethral resistance; the patient is either unaware that it is happening or, if aware, cannot control it. The term enuresis refers to incontinence, usually nocturnal, in children without detectable organic disease, and represents a persistence of an infantile pattern of bladder activity.

636 In cases of incontinence, urodynamic studies help to distinguish between increased bladder pressure (due, for example, to uninhibited detrusor contractions—the so-called unstable bladder) and reduced sphincter resistance (due to sphincter damage or weakness). These studies find a particular use in the investigation of postprostatectomy incontinence, which may be found to be due to uninhibited detrusor contractions rather than a damaged urethral sphincter.

637 Careful clinical, radiographic and urodynamic assessments are important. Depending on the aetiology, treatment may include catheterization, external appliances, urethrotomy, prostatic resection or urinary diversion. Drugs such as anticholinergics may help uninhibited detrusor contractions and occasionally electrical implants may be used to maintain sphincteric action.

638 Acute urinary retention can occur without previous urinary symptoms or may be superimposed on a progressive history of increasing urinary difficulty; it is usually painful and the bladder is distended, tense and tender. Symptomatic relief is usually immediate once the obstruction has been relieved by catheterization. In chronic retention the detrusor muscle of the bladder has become large and atonic. Huge distension may occur and the patient is usually unaware of it. Dribbling micturition and overflow incontinence are common. In addition, due to the progressive effects of obstruction on the upper urinary tracts, there may be chronic renal failure.

639 Acute retention is usually due to outflow obstruction which may be caused by benign prostatic hypertrophy, carcinoma of the prostate, urethral stricture, clot retention, vesical stones or tumours around the bladder neck. Following surgery it may occur due to a combination of pain, anaesthesia and recumbency, and in the absence of organic obstruction. Extrinsic compression from a loaded rectum, and in women a gravid or retroverted uterus or pelvic tumour, may compress the bladder outlet. Neurological causes such as spina bifida, multiple sclerosis or spinal cord tumours should not be overlooked.

640 In a patient without previous urinary symptoms adequate sedation and a warm bath may do the trick. Failing this the patient should be catheterized; often the catheter can be removed straight away and normal micturition will be re-established once the patient is mobile. If there are pre-existing urinary

difficulties then an indwelling catheter should be left for several days. If retention recurs after removal of the catheter a urologist should be consulted.

641 Bleeding may occur from veins in the wall of the bladder or from the kidney, due to reactive hyperaemia. Furthermore, a marked diuresis and natriuresis can follow, requiring intravenous replacement. Therefore, it is best to drain a chronically distended bladder slowly.

642 The risks of prolonged catheterization are urinary sepsis and urethral stricture. If the patient is in hospital there is the added risk that infection will be due to a resistant organism. To minimize these risks the softest, smallest catheter suitable for the purpose should be inserted under strictly aseptic conditions and a closed drainage system employed. For long-term use, silicone rubber catheters are less irritant.

643 Following catheterization, urine should be cultured and any infection treated. If there is evidence of renal impairment, fluid balance and anaemia should be corrected and catheter drainage continued until the patient is fit for surgery. Other investigations include an IVU and serum acid phosphatase to exclude prostatic carcinoma. A cystoscopy is always performed immediately prior to prostatectomy.

644 The size, shape and texture of the gland, and the mobility of the overlying rectal wall can be assessed. The normal adult prostate is about the size of a chestnut and has discrete lateral margins and an easily palpable median groove. The normal gland has a texture resembling the tensed thenar eminence and the overlying rectal wall is freely mobile. Hard nodules, loss of the borders and the median groove, and fixity of the rectal wall strongly suggest carcinoma, while induration and tenderness are due to inflammatory changes.

645 The changes typically occur in the central part of the gland adjacent to the urethra where there is proliferation of connective and epithelial tissues forming hyperplastic nodules. As these enlarge they compress the normal surrounding tissue into a false capsule. The connective tissue true capsule lies outside this.

646 As outflow resistance increases the detrusor muscle undergoes compensatory hypertrophy causing trabeculation, sacculation and, later, the development of diverticula and ureteric reflux. The detrusor is unable fully to overcome outflow resistance so that there is premature closure of the bladder neck, leaving

a residue of urine. Ultimately the bladder may become a chronically distended atonic bag.

647 Residual urine is likely to lead to recurrent episodes of bacterial infection.

648 Prostatectomy for benign prostatic hypertrophy is indicated when normal micturition cannot be established following acute retention; for progressive symptoms of outflow obstruction; when there is a significant amount of residual urine particularly if infected; for chronic retention with overflow; or when there are co-existent diverticula or bladder stones. Prostatectomy may also be indicated in cases of prostatic carcinoma.

649 Transurethral resection is the method of choice—this involves a piecemeal removal through an endoscope. The older suprapubic approach is not used very much these days. The aim of prostatectomy is to remove the 'adenomatous' part of the prostate whilst leaving the rim of normal compressed gland at the periphery.

650 Haemorrhage is the commonest complication. It may occur early (particularly if hypotensive anaesthesia has been used), or after 10 to 14 days, due to separation of slough from the prostatic bed. Haemorrhage may be further complicated by clot retention. Epididymitis occasionally develops, particularly if the urine was infected. Prostatic capsule or bladder can be perforated during transurethral resection and absorption of irrigant fluid into the circulation may follow. There is a small incidence of incontinence following prostatectomy.

651 Prostatic carcinoma most commonly presents with urinary symptoms indistinguishable from those of benign prostatic hypertrophy. Less common presentations are backache and paraplegia due to spinal metastases. Lymphatic obstruction can cause marked lower limb, penile and scrotal oedema. In some patients it may be an incidental finding on routine rectal examination or on histological examination of operative prostatic tissue.

652 A raised serum acid phosphatase is highly suggestive of prostatic carcinoma but is not diagnostic. The diagnosis is proven by transrectal biopsy or from prostatic tissue following transurethral resection. Skeletal survey and, more recently, bone scanning are used to establish the presence and extent of bone metastases.

653 Occult carcinoma, detected incidentally in tissue removed at prostatectomy, requires no treatment if

well-differentiated, although radiotherapy may be used in younger men. Tumours confined to the gland but causing urinary symptoms are usually treated by transurethral resection. Prostatic carcinoma is hormone responsive; stilboestrol is helpful in the control of recurrent urinary symptoms and bone pain, but seems not to alter prognosis. Because of the side-effects of stilboestrol, even in small doses, orchidectomy is often used as an alternative.

654 Even in the small doses now used (usually 1 mg t.d.s.) stilboestrol may cause fluid retention leading to ankle and pulmonary oedema. Painful gynaecomastia may be troublesome and impotence is common. There is an increased risk of deep venous thrombosis.

655 The commonest causes of urethral stricture are trauma and infection. Traumatic strictures may be due to perineal injury or pelvic fracture and usually affect the posterior urethra; sometimes they may be iatrogenic, due to catheters or instrumentation. Strictures due to gonococcal or chlamydial infection involve the penile urethra. Rarely, strictures may be congenital or malignant.

656 The urethra can be divided into penile, bulbar, membranous and prostatic parts. The bulbar urethra is vulnerable in direct perineal trauma and the membranous urethra in pelvic fractures.

657 Pelvic fractures are the cause of membranous urethral injuries, particularly when a central pubic fragment is displaced backwards. The prostate is fixed to the symphysis by the strong puboprostatic ligaments so that it moves with the bone fragment, tearing away from the membranous urethra. The patient is usually unable to pass urine, and blood is apparent at the external meatus.

658 Inexpert catheterization may complete a partial urethral tear, thus increasing the chance of severe stricture. Patients thought to have this injury should be referred for expert assessment.

The male genitalia

659 Testicular enlargement may be inflammatory, malignant or traumatic. Orchitis is painful and usually secondary to urinary infection or part of a viral illness. Tumours are typically painless. Trauma may rupture the testis and produce a traumatic haematocele.

660 Epididymo-orchitis is usually secondary to infection elsewhere in the urinary tract and is most commonly

seen in men with prostatism and infected residual urine. Gonorrhoea, and sometimes *Chlamydia*, may be the cause in younger men. Tuberculosis should be suspected in chronic epididymitis.

661 The differential diagnosis is so difficult that, in the absence of unequivocal evidence of urinary tract infection, anyone under the age of 25 with spontaneous onset of acute testicular pain and swelling should be assumed to have torsion until proven otherwise by exploration.

662 Testicular torsion usually occurs in people in whom the axis of the testis is horizontal rather than oblique; this is associated with high attachment of the tunica vaginalis to the vas and gives rise to the term 'bell clapper testis'. Sometimes there is a long 'mesentery' between the testis and epididymis so that torsion can occur within a normal tunica.

663 Urgent operation is performed—the scrotum is opened, the diagnosis confirmed and the testis untwisted. If viable, the testis is fixed in position to prevent recurrence and the opposite testis is also fixed as the underlying abnormality is often bilateral. If the torsion has been present for many hours the testis may be non-viable and is better removed.

664 Almost all testicular tumours are primary. Seminomas account for 40 per cent of cases, teratomas 30 per cent, combined tumours about 15 per cent and the rest are rarities. Teratomas are classified according to their degree of differentiation—teratoma differentiated, malignant teratoma intermediate, malignant teratoma undifferentiated and malignant teratoma trophoblastic.

665 Clinical examination is performed to assess pelvic, para-aortic and supraclavicular nodes; gynaecomastia may occasionally be present. Pulmonary metastases are looked for on chest x-ray, while CT scanning may show abdominal or mediastinal lymph node involvement. Human chorionic gonadotrophin and alpha-fetoprotein are useful serum tumour markers. Following histological confirmation by orchidectomy, IVU and lymphography are usually performed to assess nodal involvement.

666 This is performed via an inguinal approach in the belief that early control of the cord may prevent iatrogenic tumour dissemination. In addition, a scrotal approach risks contaminating a different lymphatic field.

667 Seminomas are radiosensitive and, following orchidectomy, radiotherapy to para-aortic and ipsilateral iliac nodes is given; subsequently mediastinal and supraclavicular nodes can be irradiated if involved. Five-year survival is 80 to 90 per cent. Teratomas are less radiosensitive and require higher doses; disseminated tumours are treated with intensive chemotherapy.

668 A hydrocele is a collection of fluid within the tunica vaginalis. Hydroceles often occur without underlying testicular pathology, although they may be secondary to underlying disease such as tumour or infection. It is important to exclude an underlying cause by cytological examination of the fluid and palpation of the testis after aspiration, especially if the fluid is bloody.

669 A hydrocele forms in front of the testis, filling the potential space provided by the tunica vaginalis, so that the testis may be impalpable within it.

670 Idiopathic hydroceles can be treated by aspiration, though they often reaccumulate. Excision or plication of the sac is the definitive treatment. Some surgeons advocate injection of phenol solution after aspiration to prevent recurrence. In infants, communicating hydroceles are treated by ligation of the processus vaginalis. If secondary, treatment is directed to the underlying pathology.

671 Fluid from a hydrocele is a clear golden yellow, from an epididymal cyst clear and colourless, while the fluid from a spermatocele is milky due to the presence of sperm.

672 A varicocele is a soft, lumpy mass, related to the testis, is due to varicosity of the pampiniform plexus and has been said to feel like 'a bag of worms'. It is commoner on the left than the right, may be related to the differing anatomy of testicular venous drainage on the two sides—the left testicular vein enters the left renal vein while the right drains directly into the vena cava. Very rarely a left-sided varicocele may be caused by a renal tumour growing into the renal vein and obstructing the testicular vein. Varicoceles may become large and cause discomfort. About 20 per cent of men attending infertility clinics have oligospermia associated with a varicocele—in these, ligation of the veins at the internal inguinal ring may produce a dramatic improvement in sperm counts.

673 In all but 3 per cent of full-term boys both testes are in the scrotum at birth and in all but 0.7 per cent at a

year. Thus spontaneous descent can happen up to the age of one year but is unlikely after this.

674 An undescended testis is one in which descent has been arrested at some point along the normal path, while in maldescent the testis lies outside the normal path of descent. A retractile testis is one which, due to cremasteric contraction, appears undescended but can be coaxed down with the warm examining hand.

675 An incompletely descended testis may be located retroperitoneally in the abdomen, or in the inguinal canal where it will usually be palpable. The maldescended testis usually lies in the superficial inguinal pouch, which is anterior to the external oblique aponeurosis, lateral to the external ring; rarer sites include the perineum, root of the penis and the femoral triangle.

676 Seventy per cent of undescended testes are associated with indirect inguinal hernia. There is a higher risk of torsion and trauma. Fertility is at risk if the testis is still out of the scrotum after the age of five years because both the development of tubules and spermatogenesis are delayed. The chance of malignancy is increased thirty-five-fold and this risk is reduced but not abolished by orchidopexy.

677 As spontaneous descent does not occur after the age of one, orchidopexy should be performed as soon as convenient after this and certainly by the age of five, by which time histological changes can be seen in the testis. Orchidopexy involves locating the testis, mobilizing it by dividing all its attachments apart from the vas and its blood supply and then placing and retaining it within the scrotum, usually by fashioning a dartos pouch.

678 Phimosis is narrowing of the orifice of the prepuce. It occurs predominantly in small boys, in whom it may be congenital or acquired, and old men. In small boys the normal prepuce is often not retractable until the age of four or five, thus predisposing to balanitis which may cause phimosis. In adults it is usually secondary to poor hygiene leading to balanitis. Paraphimosis occurs when a tight prepuce is drawn back over the glans and left, causing venous engorgement distal to the constriction, making simple reduction impossible.

679 Impotence is psychogenic in over 50 per cent of cases. Organic causes include diabetes, aorto-iliac atherosclerosis, damage to pelvic autonomic nerves during rectal and vascular surgery, spinal trauma and various drugs.

680 Following vasectomy it takes about 12 to 20 ejaculations to clear the system of sperms. Normally seminal analysis is performed at 12 and 16 weeks following vasectomy and the absence of motile sperms in a fresh sample indicates that vasectomy has been effective.

The heart, lungs and thoracic contents

681 The commonest problem is pain but occasionally a fractured rib may puncture the visceral pleura and cause a pneumothorax. Rib fractures hurt even with quiet breathing and the pain can become very severe with coughing. Patients with pre-existing respiratory disease, in particular bronchitics who need to cough frequently to clear their sputum, are especially at risk and can get into trouble with sputum retention, areas of pulmonary collapse and consolidation and may go into respiratory failure.

682 The term 'flail chest' is used when a group of ribs are fractured in two places so that there is a mobile panel in the chest wall, no longer adequately connected to the skeletal structure. This can occur on one side or, if there are bilateral fractures, the sternum may be part of the flail segment. As the patient expands his chest to inhale air the flail segment moves inwards paradoxically, reducing the useful inspiratory volume. If breathing is very inefficient, the only effective treatment is to use positive pressure ventilation and this may have to be started urgently with an endotracheal tube and a bag, especially if there are other injuries.

683 Any time that there is recent onset of breathlessness or even sudden deterioration in a previously breathless patient we should consider the possibility of pneumothorax. Three particular patterns can be recognized: the previously fit young person with a spontaneous pneumothorax; the injured patient with rib fractures who may suddenly deteriorate; and the chronic chest patient in sudden acute distress. The signs are reduced breath sounds and increased resonance on the side of the pneumothorax, and the trachea may be shifted away from it. An urgently performed chest x-ray will confirm the diagnosis; it is extremely unusual to have to put in a drain without this being available.

684 In tension pneumothorax air continues to escape from the lung into the pleural space but, due to a valve-like effect, the air is trapped and an increasing amount accumulates. The lung becomes completely collapsed and then, as the pressure builds up, the mediastinum

becomes displaced, venous return is impaired and a circulatory abnormality is added to the respiratory problem. The ideal treatment is with an intercostal tube connected to an underwater seal but in an emergency a wide-bore, intravenous cannula inserted through the second intercostal space will relieve the tension.

685 Any pneumothorax which is endangering life should be dealt with urgently. This includes tension pneumothorax in anybody, but in a patient with underlying lung disease, a relatively small pneumothorax may also require urgent treatment to relieve severe respiratory difficulty. A complete pneumothorax should be drained as should a lesser pneumothorax which fails to expand on conservative management. A multiply injured patient with a pneumothorax who requires a general anaesthetic should have a drain inserted to avoid tension pneumothorax developing with positive pressure ventilation. Although the traditional site for an intercostal drain is the second space anteriorly, a drain placed in the midaxillary line above the level of the nipple is safer and is least likely to damage intrathoracic structures or to end up below the diaphragm.

686 Surgical emphysema is air in the soft tissues which can be felt as crepitus. It tracks along tissue planes and is typically most marked around the neck, shoulders and the face. It implies leakage of air under some degree of pressure. It occurs with rupture of an air-containing viscus in communication with soft tissues. The commonest cause is traumatic pneumothorax where the breach in the parietal pleura caused by the same rib fracture permits air to enter the chest wall. It can also occur with spontaneous or traumatic rupture of a major airway or the oesophagus when the air tracks up from the mediastinum.

687 With an open chest wound air can be sucked freely into the pleural space on inspiration and the lung collapses away from the chest wall. Ventilation is therefore quite ineffective on that side and severely reduced in its efficiency on the other side. A non-porous dressing such as tulle gras should be applied over the wound after asking the patient to perform a Valsalva manoeuvre to expel at least some of the intrathoracic air. If the dressing is effective the patient is now at risk from tension pneumothorax so this should be looked for and can be relieved by removing and reapplying the dressing.

688 To detect the presence of free air or blood in the chest the x-ray beam has to be horizontal. The best is an x-ray

taken with the patient sitting up. If the patient's condition precludes this, a compromise such as a semi-erect film or a lateral decubitus should be considered. A supine x-ray can be falsely reassuring because both free air and blood can be missed if viewed en face.

689   The possibility that the chest will have to be opened to control haemorrhage must now be considered. A laterally placed, underwater seal drain will not only deal with the pneumothorax but will also drain blood. The bottle should be marked and the rate of bleeding measured because this information will help in deciding whether a thoracotomy is required. Blood is the most likely fluid to appear but very rarely there may be gastro-intestinal contents or chyle.

690   It is possible that he has a tear of the aorta caused by sudden deceleration. The typical site is in the descending aorta just beyond the origin of the left subclavian artery; the tear can be temporarily contained by the aortic adventitia and the overlying mediastinal pleura. An emergency anteroposterior chest x-ray can be misleading, but if an aortic tear seems at all likely, urgent aortograms should be obtained, after referral to a thoracic unit.

691   Haemoptysis can be the presenting symptom with cancer, infection or infarction of the lung. The commonest tumour that presents with this symptom is bronchial carcinoma (70 per cent present in this way) but it can occur with other tumours, benign or malignant from the larynx on down the respiratory tract. It can be part of the picture of infective conditions such as tuberculosis, bronchiectasis, pneumonia or even bronchitis but the possible co-existence of carcinoma must be remembered. Infarction due to pulmonary embolus can present this way. The nature of the accompanying sputum and the other history may help in establishing a diagnosis but it is a serious symptom and should be investigated.

692   A patient with a pleural effusion is usually breathless, the severity depending on the size of the effusion and the respiratory reserve of the patient. The percussion note is dull over the effusion and the breath sounds are very diminished or absent. In the erect chest x-ray there is opacification which extends upwards from the base in proportion to the volume of the fluid. The upper border appears to curve up laterally because the x-ray beam passes tangentially through a greater thickness of fluid. A fluid level is only seen if there is also a pneumothorax.

693 Pleural effusions occur with infections such as pneumonia and tuberculosis; malignancy, most commonly secondary from breast or ovary; heart failure; collagen diseases involving the pleura; and metabolic disease associated with reduced plasma oncotic pressure such as cirrhosis.

694 Patients with lung cancer usually present with new respiratory symptoms which include cough in 80 per cent, haemoptysis in 70 per cent and dyspnoea in 60 per cent. Pain is a relatively late feature and is part of the presentation in 40 per cent. Chance observation on chest x-ray is not infrequent but more commonly the patient has already had some symptoms leading to the request.

695 Cytological examination of sputum is a valuable, non-invasive test, but if the tumour can be reached, direct biopsy through the fibre-optic or rigid bronchoscope is the best way to make a definitive diagnosis. Peripheral tumours can be diagnosed by fine needle aspiration under x-ray control and the resulting specimen examined cytologically. For more extensive disease lymph node biopsies obtained by mediastinoscopy or direct exploration in the neck can be examined histologically.

696 Bronchial carcinoma spreads via lymphatics and in the blood. Lymphatic spread is first to the ipsilateral hilar nodes and then to the mediastinal nodes. Blood-borne spread is to the brain, bones, particularly ribs, vertebrae and proximal long bones, the liver and the adrenal glands. These may all be clinically undetectable at the time of presentation and should be deliberately sought by investigation if futile thoracotomy is to be avoided.

697 The differential diagnosis includes malignant and inflammatory diseases. Bronchial carcinoma is a common cause, in the appropriate age group, while symmetrical lymphadenopathy suggests lymphoma. Tuberculosis and sarcoid can both present in this way.

698 Myasthenia gravis and thymic tumours are indications for thymectomy. Myasthenic patients without a thymoma, in particular young women, are the most likely to get a good symptomatic result. Thymectomy is also indicated for thymoma which may be locally malignant or may result in a variety of syndromes including red cell aplasia.

699 An empyema is an abscess within the pleural space. It has thickened walls with fibrin deposited on parietal and visceral pleura and it contains pus. There is adherence of the lung to the chest wall over part of its

surface. As with all abscesses the primary management is drainage which can usually be achieved by an intercostal drain and should be followed by systemic and local antibiotics. Traditionally, an inch of a suitable rib is resected and open drainage is instigated. This old-fashioned management is inappropriate and frankly dangerous if the term 'empyema' is loosely applied to all infected pleural effusions.

700   A bronchopleural fistula is a communication between the bronchus and the pleural space and is a life threatening complication of lung resection, in particular pneumonectomy. It typically presents one to three weeks after the operation and results in air and infected material entering the pleural space, and pleural fluid sometimes suddenly and in large quantities, flooding the remaining lung. A lung abscess or cavitating carcinoma may rupture into the pleural space and produce the same effect.

701   The highest incidence of tuberculosis is in the immigrant communities, in particular from the Indian subcontinent. Those with reduced resistance due to malnutrition, alcoholism, steroid therapy or intercurrent disease are also more susceptible.

702   Thoracic vertebrae may collapse as a result of malignant invasion, infection or osteoporosis. Collapse due to malignancy is usually the result of a secondary deposit and a single vertebra is involved. Infection, most commonly due to tuberculosis, involves two adjacent vertebrae and there is a paravertebral abscess. Collapse results in wedging of the spine, squeezing out of infected material and may cause paraplegia. Osteoporotic vertebral collapse occurs in the elderly.

703   Immunosuppressed patients are at risk from otherwise unlikely organisms, in particular transplant patients and those having chemotherapy for malignant disease. *Aspergillus* can grow as an opportunistic saprophyte in old TB cavities. Primary infections are otherwise rare in Britain although in areas of the United States these diseases are endemic, particularly in the South West for coccidioidomycosis and the South East for blastomycosis and histoplasmosis.

704   Those least able to protect their airways. This includes those with a reduced level of consciousness due to alcohol, drugs, head injury or anaesthesia. Children can inhale small toys or peanuts in the course of games. Laryngeal obstruction results in death by asphyxiation if not quickly relieved. Much more

commonly the foreign body lodges more distally and, if not removed, the lung beyond it collapses and becomes infected and a lung abscess may form.

705 There is expectoration of copious amounts of foul smelling sputum, sometimes streaked with blood. There are recurrent, superimposed episodes of acute lung infection causing exacerbation of symptoms with, in addition, fever and pleuritic pain.

706 Surgery is indicated in the management of endocarditis if there is intractable cardiac failure, uncontrolled infection or if conduction defects develop, indicating septal abscess formation. In general the outlook is much better if surgery can be avoided until the infection is completely resolved but sometimes, for example, with severe valvar regurgitation, operation is the only way to control heart failure. Occasionally the organism, which may be a fungus, is so resistant to treatment that valve replacement is essential. The overall mortality for patients who require surgery for endocarditis is of the order of 50 per cent.

707 Aneurysms of the arch and descending aorta are usually atheromatous, while in the ascending aorta they may be due to syphilis or Marfan's syndrome. Dissecting aneurysms, usually due to atheroma, can involve all three parts of the thoracic aorta and are subdivided according to the site of the tear and the extent of the dissection.

708 Rupture into the pericardial sac causing tamponade or, if the dissection progresses retrogradely to the aortic root, occlusion of a coronary or acute aortic valve incompetence may result.

709 Careful control of the arterial pressure, observation for symptoms and signs of extension and aortography to diagnose involvement of the ascending aorta are important parts of the management of aortic dissections. Dissections confined to the descending aorta do as well with conservative treatment as with surgery. Involvement of the ascending aorta is an indication for early surgery.

710 The head and neck vessels may become occluded with aneurysms involving the arch causing ischaemic cerebral damage. The spinal cord receives part of its blood supply from the descending aorta and the adequacy of collaterals is unpredictable. These complications may be a result of the pathology, investigation or surgical treatment and so should be looked for regularly during management.

711 Infection, heart failure and the development of
pulmonary hypertension are possible but not inevitable
consequences of the ductus remaining open. As with
other congenital heart lesions the patient is at risk from
infection which in this instance is an endarteritis of the
pulmonary artery. The risk of heart failure depends on
the size of the left to right shunt. Pulmonary
hypertension with reversal of the shunt may result and
this is known as Eisenmenger's syndrome and
precludes surgical closure. The tendency of the duct to
calcify is an additional and surgically important
consequence.

712 The clinical findings are a reduction in volume and a
delay in the femoral pulses compared with radials and
upper limb hypertension. There is a systolic murmur
and sometimes a continuous hum, both heard best at the
back. The narrowed segment of the aorta is just beyond
the origin of the left subclavian and this obstruction
causes the changes in the femoral pulses and the
systolic murmur. Flow in collaterals is responsible for
the hum and the proximal hypertension is due to a renal
response to reduced pressure below the coarctation. On
chest x-ray the '3-sign' is typically seen due to
prominence of the left subclavian above and a post
stenotic dilatation below the coarctation. The ribs from
the third downwards are irregularly notched along
their lower borders due to the enlargement of the
intercostal arteries carrying blood from the internal
mammary artery to the aorta below the coarctation.

713 The four features are pulmonary stenosis, a high
ventricular septal defect, overriding of the aorta and
right ventricular hypertrophy.

714 Mitral stenosis can be relieved by closed mitral
valvotomy, or by open valvotomy performed on by-pass.
Regurgitation is usually corrected by valve
replacement although it is sometimes possible to repair
the valve.

715 Thrombo-embolic complications, endocarditis and
valve failure may occur at any time after valve
replacement. The mechanical valves are more prone to
thrombus formation which may obstruct the valve
mechanism or be thrown off as emboli, so all patients
must be anticoagulated. Endocarditis occurs with tissue
and mechanical valves, so all dental procedures should
be preceded by antibiotic prophylaxis. Valve failure
tends to be slow but inevitable with tissue valves and is
less common but sudden and disastrous with
mechanical valves.

716 The history may include syncopal attacks, angina,
breathlessness on exertion and fatigue, but many

patients are asymptomatic. The pulse is slow-rising and there is an ejection systolic murmur heard best at the base which radiates into the neck.

717 Coronary artery by-pass grafting is indicated for the symptomatic relief of angina; it also improves the prognosis in certain categories of coronary artery disease. Patients with angina not readily controlled by medical treatment, and severe enough to interfere with a reasonable life style, should be considered for surgery, because symptomatic relief can be obtained in about 90 per cent. A strongly positive exercise ECG, whatever the degree of angina, is an indication for angiography with a view to surgery.

718 Prognosis is improved with surgery in left main stem coronary artery stenosis from about 70 per cent to about 85 per cent five-year survival, and in three vessel coronary artery disease from about 80 per cent to about 95 per cent five-year survival. Patients with impaired left ventricular function also have an improved prognosis with surgery. In fact in all but the benign forms of the disease where prognosis is good in any case, revascularization improves the chances of survival.

719 Angina pectoris means a choking sensation in the chest, from the Latin 'angere' to choke, and is the way patients frequently describe their symptom. Ludwig's angina is cellulitis of the floor of the mouth. In Vincent's angina a pseudomembrane forms on the pharynx and tonsils and two organisms (the spirochaete, *Borrelia vincenti* and a fusiform bacillus) are typically found.

720 Acute mitral regurgitation due to papillary muscle infarction and acute ventricular septal defect due to rupture of a septal infarct can both be surgically corrected. These operations have a high mortality and are only performed if the patient's outlook is hopeless without surgery.

721 A pacemaker system consists of an electrode in the heart muscle and a battery-driven pulse generator placed subcutaneously. The commonest arrangement is an endocardial system placed transvenously under local anaesthetic into the endocardial surface of the right ventricle. The alternative is an epicardial electrode placed surgically on the surface of either ventricle.

Neurosurgery

722 Yes. Intracranial tumours often present with late onset epilepsy. In this age group ischaemia and tumour are

the commonest causes. Normal clinical examination and skull x-ray do not exclude a tumour and investigation is essential to ensure that a remediable pathology is not present.

723 Severe headache and neck stiffness suggest meningism resulting from either subarachnoid blood or infection. The mode of onset of the patient's symptoms is important in determining the cause. Subarachnoid haemorrhage occurs instantly, whereas meningitis is of more gradual onset. Subarachnoid haemorrhage may cause a transient loss of consciousness. History of prodromal illness may precede a viral meningitis. If the infection is bacterial the patient may have symptoms of a source such as ear or sinus infection.

724 Difficulty in walking and micturition suggest a spinal lesion. In this age group metastatic extradural cord compression is the most likely cause, usually from lung, prostate or kidney. In the female, breast carcinoma is the most common primary site.

725 Vertebral tenderness, a sensory loss corresponding to the site of the lesion and paraparesis progressing to paraplegia support a diagnosis of cord compression. A large bladder and a lax anal sphincter indicate concomitant autonomic dysfunction.

726 Yes. The presence of a skull fracture in a conscious patient increases the risk of an intracranial haematoma 400 times. Hospital admission should allow earlier detection of a traumatic haematoma, thus reducing the chance of secondary brain damage, that is, brain damage occurring secondarily to damage at impact.

727 Basal skull fractures are difficult to spot on x-ray. Clinical evidence includes CSF rhinorrhoea or otorrhoea, periorbital haematoma, subconjunctival haemorrhage and bruising over the mastoid; of patients with these features only a half show abnormalities on skull x-ray. Detection of a basal skull fracture is important since it indicates a possible dural tear and a potential source of intracranial infection.

728 Conscious level and pupil reaction to light are the most important features to assess in a head-injured patient. Evidence of limb weakness is also relevant. A single assessment is of limited value. Repeated assessments over a few hours on the other hand are valuable in demonstrating the trend in the patient's condition.

729 The clinician must assess the patient's eye opening, verbal response and motor response and describe the patient's conscious level in these terms rather than

using vague terminology such as stupor, semicoma and coma. Eye opening occurs either spontaneously, to speech, to painful stimuli or is absent. The patient may give an orientated or confused verbal response, may utter either single words or incomprehensible sounds or have no verbal response. The optimum motor response is obeying commands. If the patient fails to respond, the examiner applies a painful stimulus to the supraorbital nerve or nail bed and observes the response in the patient's upper limbs. The patient may localize, flex, extend or have no motor response. These responses are listed in an order directly relating to worsening levels of consciousness; thus, at best, the comatose patient localizes to painful stimuli, while at worst he has no motor response.

730 Pupil dilatation and failure to react to light suggest a third nerve palsy and are useful localizing signs as they always occur on the side of the expanding lesion. There is midline shift initially, followed by herniation of the medial edge of the temporal lobe through the tentorial hiatus. This herniation compresses not only the third nerve but also the mid-brain. Local damage to the eye may also result in a fixed dilated pupil.

731 Limb weakness is detected by observing the response of the limbs to painful stimuli. Any inequality in the response on each side indicates a weakness on the side of the poorer response. Thus, localization of the left arm to pain and flexion of the right arm indicates a right-sided weakness. Alternatively, flexion in the right arm and extension in the left indicates a weakness of the left side.

732 A skull x-ray is the first line investigation, but a CT scan is necessary to indicate the exact site, nature and size of an intracranial haematoma.

733 The most commonly found lesion is a mixture of subdural and intracerebral haematoma where the latter has burst out on to the cortical surface of the frontal or temporal lobes, i.e., a 'burst' lobe (35 per cent). Approximately 20 per cent of intracranial haematomas are pure subdurals and a further 20 per cent discrete intracerebral haematomas. Extradural haematomas occur in about 15 per cent of cases, the remainder being made up of mixed extradural and intradural lesions.

734 A fracture running across the line of the middle meningeal artery may tear this vessel and cause an extradural haemorrhage. Less commonly, extradural bleeding can result from fractures crossing the sagittal or transverse sinus.

735 Shearing damage to the white matter, due to movement of the brain within the skull on deceleration, is a common contributory cause of coma in patients without intracranial haematoma. This may range from a mild injury causing transient loss of consciousness to a severe and fatal injury. Other factors include diffuse hypoxic damage, or tentorial and tonsillar herniation from diffuse cerebral swelling. Cortical contusions or lacerations, the common precursors of intradural bleeding, do not in themselves contribute to depression of conscious level.

736 Space-occupying traumatic haematomas require urgent evacuation through a craniotomy (a large bone flap). In exceptional circumstances, where speed is essential, burr hole decompression of an extradural haematoma may halt a rapid deterioration in conscious level, but in general, burr hole exploration outside a neurosurgical unit is not advised.

737 Chronic subdural haematoma occurs usually in infancy or in the elderly tending to cause a gradual deterioration in conscious level often with a fluctuating course, although focal signs may also occur. Chronic subdural haematomas may not present until several months after injury and in some patients no history of head injury is obtained.

738 After approximately 14 days subdural collections liquefy and are easily evacuated through burr holes. A subdural drain may be left in place. In a proportion of patients re-collection occurs and re-evacuation is required. Subdural peritoneal shunting or craniotomy are rarely necessary.

739 Yes. In this situation mere suture of the laceration would produce considerable risk of meningitis or cerebral abscess formation. The wound must be debrided, the depressed bone fragments elevated and either removed or cleaned thoroughly and returned to place. If the dura is torn and the cortical surface is lacerated the risk of epilepsy is high and prophylactic anticonvulsants are given.

740 A rise in intracranial pressure causes headache, usually worse in the mornings and aggravated by coughing or stooping. Vomiting may occur, often without warning. Examination of the optic fundus may reveal papilloedema. Since tumour expansion is slow, considerable compensation is possible, but eventually the patient's conscious level will deteriorate.

741 In children, suture diastasis (especially the coronal suture) is clear evidence of raised intracranial pressure. The 'beaten brass' appearance due to

increased convolutional markings, sometimes thought
to signify raised intracranial pressure, is of little help
since it often occurs in normal children. In adults and
older children, erosion of the dorsum sella is a
significant indicant of raised intracranial pressure,
although a local suprasellar lesion such as
craniopharyngioma can produce similar changes.

742 If intracranial tumour is suspected from clinical
findings, referral to a specialist unit must be arranged.
(a) Preliminary investigations carried out in the
general hospital must include a chest x-ray to help
exclude a lung primary; skull x-ray may show pineal
shift, evidence of raised intracranial pressure, bony
erosion or tumour calcification. An EEG may
demonstrate a focus and aid localization. Isotope
scanning is a useful screening test. In view of the risk
of precipitating tentorial or tonsillar herniation,
lumbar puncture is not advised. (b) In a
neurology/neurosurgical unit the investigation of
choice is the CT scan. This demonstrates the site of the
lesion and when repeated after intravenous contrast
injection often indicates its nature. Angiography is
sometimes of value in showing abnormal tumour
circulation and in demonstrating the exact
relationship or involvement of blood vessels.

743 In adults the commonest intracranial tumour is
metastatic. Of the primary cerebral tumours,
astrocytoma occurs most frequently, usually the poorly
differentiated anaplastic type. In children,
supratentorial tumours are rare. The commonest
tumour is the cerebellar medulloblastoma.

744 Yes. It is necessary to confirm the diagnosis and this
cannot be done on CT scan. Otherwise cerebral abscess
or a highly radiosensitive tumour such as lymphoma
may be missed. Burr hole biopsy is usually sufficient to
identify the lesion. In patients with malignant glioma,
open craniotomy and tumour decompression increases
mean survival by only a few months so this is usually
reserved for more benign types of tumour.

745 A parasagittal meningioma at the level of the
precentral gyrus may cause bilateral cortical damage.
If this selectively affects the medial/superior
portion of the motor strip, leg weakness is produced.

746 Yes, but this depends on the site of origin. A 'complete'
removal must include the point of dural attachment.
This is seldom possible when the meningioma arises
from the skull base, the transverse sinus or the
posterior two-thirds of the sagittal sinus. Incomplete
removal greatly increases the chance of recurrence.

747 Acoustic neuromas are associated with this familial disease. They present with a progressive deafness. Patients may also experience transient bouts of vertigo and tinnitus but these are seldom prominent features. With further growth cerebellar signs develop followed by aqueduct compression and hydrocephalus. Other cranial nerve palsies (especially the 5th nerve) may occur, but the 7th cranial nerve is remarkably resilient to damage despite its close relationship to the tumour.

748 Recent immunoassay techniques permit a classification based on the hormone type secreted—prolactinoma, GH secreting tumour and ACTH secreting tumour. (TSH and FSH/LH secreting tumours are extremely rare.) This supersedes the old classification of pituitary tumours, based on histological staining characteristics—acidophil, basophil and chromophobe adenoma.

749 Suprasellar extension of a pituitary adenoma causes compression of the optic chiasma, producing a superior bitemporal quadrantanopia initially, progressing to a bitemporal hemianopia.

750 The operative approach to the pituitary fossa is from above via a subfrontal route or from below via either a transphenoidal or transethmoidal route. Approaches from below carry a low risk and are now most frequently used. Some tumours with large lateral or anterior suprasellar extension require a subfrontal approach to permit adequate exposure and tumour removal.

751 If there is no papilloedema, lumbar puncture can be performed and reveals uniformly blood stained CSF with a xanthochromic supernatant. If papilloedema is present, then CT scan usually confirms the diagnosis, showing blood (areas of increased density) in the basal cisterns and interhemispheric or Sylvian fissures.

752 Arteriovenous malformation, tumour, anticoagulant treatment or a bleeding diathesis may cause subarachnoid haemorrhage. However, in approximately 30 per cent of patients even after four-vessel angiography the cause will not have been discovered.

753 Expansion or rupture of an aneurysm arising from the origin of the posterior communicating artery (or occasionally from the basilar bifurcation) may cause a third nerve palsy due to direct pressure.

754 A CT scan usually confirms the presence of subarachnoid blood and by demonstrating a focal collection may indicate the exact site of the ruptured

aneurysm. This is especially useful if multiple aneurysms are present. Irrespective of the CT scan findings, angiography is required to determine and delineate the exact nature of the lesion.

755 About 60 per cent of patients survive the initial aneurysm rupture but subsequent mortality risks are high. The aneurysm may rebleed, causing death in two out of three patients. The rebleed risk diminishes with time but never disappears. Breakdown products of blood in contact with the intracranial vessels cause vasospasm in 50 per cent of patients and many develop clinical evidence of cerebral ischaemia. Finally the presence of blood in the CSF may block its normal route of absorption at the arachnoid villi causing a communicating hydrocephalus.

756 (a) In the first six months approximately 40 per cent of survivors of the initial aneurysm rupture rebleed; of these two-thirds die.
(b) Beyond the first six months after aneurysm rupture, the risk of rebleeding is 3.5 per cent per year; again two-thirds of the patients rebleeding die. Thus the risk of death from rebleeding after the first six months is 25 per cent over a 10-year period.

757 Clipping of the aneurysm neck at operation is the only certain way of preventing rebleeding. Antifibrinolytic drugs are often given with the theoretical aim of preventing clot resorption around the aneurysm fundus. Their benefit however in reducing the rebleed rate has yet to be proven. Reactive hypertension commonly occurs after subarachnoid haemorrhage and often antihypertensives are administered. Again their benefit in reducing the rebleed rate is not certain, and reduction of blood pressure in patients with impaired autoregulation (as occurs after subarachnoid haemorrhage) may exacerbate any pre-existing cerebral ischaemia.

758 Arteriovenous malformations usually present with subarachnoid haemorrhage (78 per cent), but 16 per cent of patients present with epilepsy. In a few, focal signs or signs of raised intracranial pressure predominate.

759 Straight spinal x-rays in a patient with metastatic cord compression may show erosion of the pedicle, collapse or erosion of the vertebral body or a paravertebral mass. These features should correspond with the patient's sensory level. If not, multiple lesions must be considered.

760 Tumours, infective and degenerative lesions are the main benign causes of cord compression. Tumours include neurofibroma, meningioma, lipoma and dermoid/epidermoid cysts. Infective lesions may be acute staphylococcal or chronic tuberculous. Cord compression from osteo-arthritic degeneration usually occurs in the cervical spine. Rarely, acute disc protrusion and angiomatous malformation may present in this manner.

761 A lateral disc protrusion at L5/S1 level usually compresses the S1 nerve root. This causes leg pain radiating down to the lateral aspect of the foot or sole. The pain is typically aggravated by coughing or straining. Signs of S1 root compression include weakness of the plantar flexors and invertors of the foot, impaired sensation over the lateral border of the foot and a diminished or absent ankle jerk. A straight leg raising deficit will almost certainly be noted but this is not specific for any one root.

762 Hydrocephalus means an increase in cerebrospinal fluid (CSF) volume within the skull. CSF is secreted by the choroid plexus, which passes out of the ventricular system through the foramina of the fourth ventricle, flows around the cerebellar and cerebral surface to be absorbed into the venous system through the arachnoid villi. A block of CSF flow at any point throughout its pathway or impaired reabsorption results in hydrocephalus. A block to flow may be caused by occlusion or narrowing of the foramen of Munro, the aqueduct of Sylvius or the fourth ventricle. This may result from tumour, congenital defect, haematoma or inflammatory exudate. Obstruction to reabsorption at the arachnoid villi is usually caused by subarachnoid haemorrhage or meningitis. Rarely hydrocephalus is caused by excessive CSF secretion from a choroid plexus papilloma.

763 Patients with symptoms of raised intracranial pressure due to hydrocephalus require a shunt. Surgeons use ventriculo-atrial or ventriculo–peritoneal shunts depending on individual preference. These incorporate a valve system to prevent an excessive reduction in CSF pressure.

764 Harvey Cushing was a pioneer in neurosurgery working in Boston at the beginning of the century. He is recognized not only for his descriptions of pituitary disease, but also for his numerous advances in neurosurgical technique.

Ear, nose and throat

765 A careful history often gives a clue. For example,
difficulty in distinguishing spoken words, especially
when there is background noise, or intolerence of
loud sounds are typical of perceptive deafness. On
the other hand, deafness following direct trauma to
the ear is usually predominantly conductive. General
clinical examination may reveal other abnormalities
sometimes associated with specific varieties of
deafness, e.g. neurofibromatosis (perceptive) or
osteogenesis imperfecta (conductive). Abnormalities
of the external auditory canal or tympanic
membrane, such as wax or a perforation, will nearly
always be visible when the deafness is conductive
and are less often seen with perceptive deafness. The
Rinne and Weber tuning fork tests should always be
done and when properly carried out are remarkably
accurate at distinguishing conductive from perceptive
hearing loss.

766 Prepare a clean aural syringe and about 200 ml of
clean water at body temperature. Before proceeding,
always ask the patient if he has had a perforated
tympanic membrane or trouble resulting from
syringing in the past—if in doubt do not proceed.
Drape a towel over the patient's shoulder and ask
him to hold a bowl to collect the water. Gently
pulling the ear upwards and backwards with one
hand, the nozzle of the syringe is just introduced into
the external auditory canal with the other and the
jet of water directed slightly upwards and forwards.
When all the wax has been removed, the ear canal
and tympanic membrane should be checked once
more. If the procedure is painful or the wax shows no
sign of moving, do not persist: instead, refer the
patient to an ENT surgeon. Complications resulting
from incorrect aural syringing are a common cause of
medicolegal complaints.

767 A swab should always be taken at the first visit and
culture for fungi as well as bacteria requested. The
mainstays of treatment are to keep the ear dry, to
remove thoroughly all debris or discharge (either
with cotton wool or a fine sucker) and to instil the
appropriate antibiotics or antifungal agents.
Systemic antibiotics are usually only used when a
furuncle is present or when the patient is diabetic.
Otitis externa complicating diabetes mellitus may be
very severe, even fatal, and is often due to
Pseudomonas species. Good diabetic control is
essential and should be combined with systemic

antibiotics, usually an aminoglycoside such as gentamicin.

768   If the discharge from the ear contains mucus, otitis media with a perforation is almost certainly present and characteristically, with an acute otitis media the pain disappears with the onset of discharge and there is no tenderness of the pinna or external auditory canal. In contrast the purulent discharge of otitis externa is never mucoid and the pinna and external auditory canal may be very painful to the touch or on chewing. Deafness is an early feature in otitis media which frequently follows an upper respiratory tract infection, whereas deafness is not present, or is a late feature, in otitis externa. If the discharge can be cleared from the external auditory canal sufficiently to allow a view of the tympanic membrane, otitis media with a purulent discharge will always be associated with a perforation, in otitis externa the membrane is usually intact.

769   'Glue ear' (more correctly called secretory otitis media) is a condition in which fluid accumulates in the middle ear space because of a partial vacuum, the cause of which is a failure of the Eustachian tube to ventilate the middle ear adequately. This happens most frequently in children, and commonly causes hearing loss. Eustachian tube malfunction occurs with adenoid hypertrophy, upper respiratory tract infections, nasal allergy and polyps, cleft-palate, and tumours of the nasopharynx.

770   The organisms most frequently cultured in acute otitis media are *Str. pneumoniae, Haemophilus influenzae*, beta-haemolytic *Streptococci* and *Staph. pyogenes. E. coli, Proteus* and *Pseudomonas* are also encountered. Viruses probably also cause acute otitis media but they are difficult to identify.

771   The history is often characteristic. In safe (tubotympanic) chronic suppurative otitis media there are recurring episodes of mucoid or mucopurulent ear discharge, usually accompanying colds or 'flu, and associated with mild or moderate loss of hearing. In the unsafe (attico-antral) type there is often a history of constant and long-standing, foul smelling ear discharge associated with a more severe deafness. The distinction can usually be made for certain on otoscopic examination. In unsafe ear disease, there is a perforation of the tympanic membrane, either in the attic or posterior marginal region and cholesteatoma is often visible. In safe ear disease, the tympanic perforation is central and cholesteatoma is absent. Audiometry will usually confirm a more severe

hearing loss in unsafe ear disease and plain x-rays and tomograms of the mastoids show sclerosis and sometimes bone erosion due to cholesteatoma. In safe ear disease, the mastoid is often pneumatized and there is no bone erosion.

772 The complications of long-standing, chronic, suppurative otitis media are due to erosion of bone and spread of disease to neighbouring structures. Erosion of bone by infection may lead to an extradural or subdural abscess. Extension superiorly gives rise to meningitis and temporal lobe abscess, and posterior extension may cause thrombosis or septic thrombophlebitis of the lateral sinus, septicaemia or a cerebellar abscess. There may be paralysis of the seventh nerve, and erosion of bone medially leading to suppurative labyrinthitis and total loss of auditory and vestibular function. This may extend to involve the apex of the petrous temporal bone (petrositis) and lead to a sixth nerve palsy and facial pain.

773 In otosclerosis, a focus of new bone formation encroaches upon the stapes footplate and prevents it from moving. The cause is unknown, although there is a variable genetic inheritance. Usually both ears are affected and it is thought that hormonal changes influence the new bone growth. For this reason women are affected more severely than men, especially if they have borne children. The deafness, which is conductive, starts early in adult life and is slowly progressive, although it never becomes total. So, in its classical form, otosclerosis presents as bilateral deafness in a young female with children, there is a family history of deafness, and clinical examination of the ears reveals no abnormality apart from a pure conductive hearing loss.

774 The symptoms of Menière's disease are deafness, tinnitus, vertigo and a feeling of pressure in the ear. One or both ears may be affected. The characteristic feature of the disease is the episodic nature of the symptoms—they may come and go in a marked and unpredictable fashion, but with an overall tendency towards deterioration over many years. The cause of the disease is not really understood and no medical treatment has ever been shown to be curative.

775 Bell's palsy is the name given to idiopathic facial paralysis. Neither the history of onset nor clinical examination give any clue as to the aetiology. A viral infection has often been suspected but never convincingly proven. The prognosis for recovery depends on the severity of the paralysis. When some movement is preserved, full recovery can be expected.

However, when the paralysis is complete 50 per cent will recover but in the remainder some permanent deformity may persist. Steroids are often given if the patient is seen within five days of the onset of paralysis but their value is unproven and they are not indicated when the paralysis is incomplete. When the cornea is exposed it should be protected with artificial tears and a tarsorrhaphy considered if there is a risk of ulceration.

776 Although many patients with tinnitus have nothing seriously wrong with them, it is a common symptom and it may be very distressing. A search should always be made for a treatable cause. At the least, this means an examination of the ears and testing the hearing with a tuning fork and by pure tone audiometry. If the tinnitus is also audible to the examiner (so called objective tinnitus) there is always a local cause, often of a vascular nature. Many common ear diseases, such as otitis media or otosclerosis, present with tinnitus, and treatment may stand a good chance of bringing relief.

777 Presbyacusis means deafness due to ageing and is due to degenerative changes in the auditory pathway. Characteristically, the hearing is worse for high frequency sounds and this causes difficulty in hearing the consonants of speech. The result is that although the patient can hear that someone is speaking, he has difficulty in distinguishing the words. When a hearing aid is used, low frequency vowel sounds are often boosted to an uncomfortable level and this may make the use of a hearing aid unacceptable.

778 Whether or not a fracture can be demonstrated on a skull x-ray following head trauma, the presence of a CSF leak from the ear indicates that a fracture of the skull base is present. Prophylactic antibiotics should be given, for example benzyl-penicillin and sulphadimidine, because of the risk of meningitis. The patient should be nursed sitting up, if possible, to lower CSF pressure. A piece of sterile cotton wool can be placed in the external auditory meatus to soak up blood and CSF but otherwise the ear should be left strictly alone. Usually the CSF leak will stop spontaneously, but if it persists for more than 10 to 14 days a neurosurgical opinion should be sought to consider surgical closure of the dural tear.

779 Many broken noses are due to assault and careful records are important for possible medicolegal use later. The first step is to take a history and carry out a thorough examination to exclude other injuries, in particular associated fractures of the facial skeleton. If

there are other injuries requiring urgent treatment, the nasal injury is of less immediate concern. First aid will usually control the epistaxis which follows a broken nose and lacerations are treated by toilet and suture as necessary. The septum should be checked for the presence of a haematoma (which requires early drainage, under general anaesthesia, if present) and x-rays of the nasal bones and facial skeleton should be taken. Bruising and swelling often prevent a full assessment of any deformity and the nose should be re-examined after five to seven days. Significant displacement with cosmetic deformity will require manipulation within fourteen days of the injury. If there is no visible displacement, manipulation is unnecessary.

780 The causes of nose bleeds are usually classified as local and general: the commonest local cause is exposed vessels in Little's area which are easily traumatized by children who pick at their noses. Repeated nose blowing because of colds often causes bleeding from the same region. Direct trauma to the nose, especially if a fracture is present, usually causes bleeding which stops spontaneously. Benign or malignant tumours in the nose are uncommon but may give rise to repeated minor epistaxes. Hereditary telangiectasia (Osler-Weber-Rendu disease) is also uncommon but almost always associated with nose bleeds. Of the general causes, systemic hypertension associated with atherosclerosis is far and away the most common. Diseases of the blood (factor and platelet deficiencies) also sometimes give rise to nose bleeds.

781 Treatment for nose bleeds is directed at correcting the underlying cause, such as hypertension, and arresting the haemorrhage. For minor nose bleeds which arise from Little's area, such as occur in children, first aid measures (sit up, lean forward, pinch the nose and breathe through the mouth) and sometimes cautery to the bleeding point with a silver nitrate stick are sufficient. For adults, especially when the bleeding point is posterior and inaccessible, some form of packing is often necessary—either anterior with ribbon gauze soaked in topical antiseptic (such as Bismuth-Iodine-Paraffin paste) or posterior with a balloon catheter. Admission to hospital for bed rest, sedation and occasionally blood transfusion is then necessary. As a last resort, the maxillary or ethmoid artery may have to be ligated surgically.

782 Infections, particularly the common cold, invariably cause some degree of nasal obstruction. Vasomotor disturbances of the nasal mucosa, both allergic (hay fever) and non-allergic, are potent causes especially

when vasoconstrictor sprays have been used repeatedly (rhinitis medicamentosa). Nasal polyps usually present with this symptom. Trauma may cause nasal obstruction which is reversible if due to mucosal swelling, but may be permanent if there is a deflection of the septum or organized septal haematoma. Large adenoids in young children and benign or malignant tumours in adults, and congenital choanal atresia complete the list.

783 When used in short sharp courses of not more than 7 to 10 days, vasoconstrictor nasal sprays do no harm. However, prolonged and frequent use may lead to habituation and the long-term consequences can be very troublesome. Eventually the vasoconstrictors in the spray cause increased permeability of the vessel walls and constant mucosal oedema (rhinitis medicamentosa). The symptoms of obstruction and watery discharge which result, will never clear up until the habit has been broken.

784 This is an operation to correct septal deformity which may be congenital or traumatic. It entails elevating the nasal lining from both sides of the bony and cartilaginous septum, and then removing or repositioning the deviated portion. The nasal lining is then allowed to come together in the mid-line and is usually held in place by a pressure pack in the nose for 24 hours.

785 Nasal allergy, which may be seasonal (hay fever) or perennial (for example dust allergy) is predominantly a Type 1 immediate hypersensitivity reaction mediated by IgE. The symptoms of nasal obstruction and discharge result from increased vessel permeability and oedema. This is caused by the release of histamine and other vaso-active substances from mast cells, as a result of the interaction between antigen and IgE.

786 Sinusitis is an infection and vasomotor rhinitis is not. A purulent discharge from the nose is characteristic of sinusitis and the appropriate antibiotic will usually help. Vasomotor rhinitis, on the other hand, is a disturbance of the vasculature in the nasal lining and any discharge is clear and watery and antibiotics make no difference to the symptoms.

787 The treatment of sinusitis may be medical or surgical. Medical treatment entails identifying the causative organism with a nasal swab, aiding sinus drainage by the use of decongestant nose drops (such as Ephedrine), loosening secretions by the inhalation of steam and treating the infection with appropriate antibiotics. If

an adequate trial of medical treatment fails to clear the
infection, then an antral puncture and washout will
often help by removing secretions and by obtaining a
further specimen for culture. Formal surgical
treatment is reserved for emergencies and failed
medical treatment. Chronic maxillary sinusitis may be
helped by making a large surgical opening for drainage
into the nose (intranasal antrostomy). A similar
drainage procedure is sometimes necessary for chronic
infections in the frontal sinus. Acute infections of the
frontal and ethmoid sinuses may lead to orbital
cellulitis and a subperiosteal abscess requiring incision
and drainage. In general, the advent of antibiotics has
reduced the need to treat sinus infection surgically.

788 The paranasal sinuses are air spaces within bone. Most
malignant tumours arise from the epithelium lining the
sinuses and symptoms do not develop until the growth
has filled the bony cavity and extended through the
bone to involve neighbouring structures. This means
that they present late, and usually only when local
infiltration has taken place. The location of the nasal
sinuses, close to the orbit and skull base, makes radical
surgical removal difficult in many cases and
unfortunately, the results of radiotherapy (the only real
alternative to surgery) are equally poor.

789 Tonsillitis, glandular fever, diphtheria, Vincent's
angina and thrush. The purulent exudate associated
with acute tonsillitis may become confluent to form a
membrane. A blood film and Paul-Bunnell test are
required to differentiate this from the similar
appearance of the tonsillitis which often accompanies
glandular fever. Diphtheria and Vincent's angina are
both rare nowadays and may both be associated with an
adherent grey membrane on the tonsils. The membrane
of oral candidiasis (thrush) is white and usually more
widespread.

790 Adenoidectomy is indicated when the adenoids are
sufficiently large to cause persistent nasal obstruction
and/or recurrent otitis media. Nasal obstruction
alone may be sufficient reason for adenoidectomy when
it is associated with recurrent upper respiratory tract
infections, rhinorrhoea and difficulty eating meals due
to the need to breathe through the mouth. When
adenoid hypertrophy is associated with Eustachian
tube obstruction and middle ear effusion or otitis media,
and there has been no response to medical treatment,
most otolaryngologists recommend adenoidectomy.

791 Nearly half of all patients with nasopharyngeal cancer
present with a symptomless lump in the neck as a result
of cervical node metastasis. If the Eustachian tube is

obstructed, then there may be a complaint of deafness because of middle ear fluid. Facial pain and double vision result from direct upward extension into the skull base with involvement of the fifth and sixth cranial nerves. Nose bleeds may occur and be associated with nasal obstruction and 'catarrh'.

792 Aphthous ulcers are common and often occur on the lateral borders or undersurface of the tongue where they may be multiple. Trauma to the tongue, whether accidental, or due to prominent teeth or an ill fitting denture, may also lead to ulceration. Malignancy should always be suspected when an ulcer shows no sign of healing after six weeks and a biopsy is essential. Other causes of tongue ulcers include herpes virus infection and local manifestations of systemic diseases such as lichen planus, blood dyscrasia, Stevens-Johnson Syndrome, vitamin deficiency and drug reaction (including Epanutin).

793 The Latin word globus means a sphere or ball and the term globus sensation is used to describe the common complaint of a feeling of a 'lump in the throat', usually at laryngeal level. The symptom is usually most noticeable between meals and may be relieved by eating. True difficulty in swallowing is absent. Although serious underlying disease is rare, a haemoglobin estimation and barium swallow should be carried out to exclude such conditions as the Patterson-Brown-Kelly syndrome, a pharyngeal pouch or carcinoma of the pharynx or upper oesophagus.

794 A pharyngeal pouch causes a rather vague difficulty in swallowing associated with regurgitation of food. When the pouch is large and laryngeal overspill has been occurring, there may also be repeated chest infections. Physical examination, including indirect laryngoscopy, rarely reveals anything. A barium swallow with AP and lateral views of the neck and thoracic inlet, is diagnostic. Endoscopic examination will confirm the diagnosis but care must be taken because of the danger of perforating the wall of the pouch with the endoscope.

795 The Patterson-Brown-Kelly syndrome is dysphagia associated with glossitis, stomatitis and iron deficiency anaemia, usually in women. If untreated, there is a definite risk of malignant change in the pharyngeal mucosa. Correction of the anaemia will usually relieve the symptoms and reduce the risk of malignancy.

796 After six weeks at the latest. Although malignant disease of the larynx as a cause of hoarseness is uncommon by comparison with laryngitis or vocal

abuse, early diagnosis is essential. Laryngoscopic examination is quick and easy to perform and the great majority of serious laryngeal diseases are visible. The cure rate for early cancers of the vocal cord is in the region of 90 per cent, whereas the five-year survival for advanced lesions, particularly if there are lymph node metastases, may be 25 per cent at best.

797   In general a lesion obstructing the airway at laryngeal level will cause inspiratory stridor. If the lesion is in the trachea, the noise will be heard equally in inspiration and expiration, while airway obstruction below this level predominantly causes expiratory wheeze.

798   Epiglottitis is an infection of the epiglottis and supralaryngeal structures, usually occurring in children, with an acute onset and very rapid progression leading to severe airway obstruction. The time taken from onset to the development of stridor may be only a few hours and there is usually a high pyrexia and marked general malaise. *Haemophilus influenzae* is the most common organism responsible for the infection. Swabs and blood cultures should be taken and treatment consists of antibiotics (chloramphenicol is often used) and the relief of airway obstruction, either by tracheostomy or intubation. Steroids may be used to reduce inflammatory oedema.

799   The commonest causes of unilateral vocal cord paralysis are carcinoma of the bronchus involving the left recurrent laryngeal nerve, trauma during thyroid surgery and an idiopathic mononeuropathy. Other causes include bulbar palsy, and carcinomas of the thyroid and oesophagus.

800   The treatment of laryngeal cancer is general and local. General measures include the correction of anaemia and nutritional deficiencies and treatment for chest infections. Local treatment may be curative or palliative. In the UK and Europe almost all laryngeal cancers are treated by radiotherapy in the first instance, to a maximum tolerated dose in an attempt to cure. Surgery is reserved for those patients who have received radiotherapy and in whom a biopsy has shown the presence of persistent or recurrent disease. Although removal of only part of the larynx is occasionally possible, surgery for most patients means a total laryngectomy. For those unfit for surgery or in whom only palliation is possible, chemotherapy or cryosurgery occasionally help. If the tumour gives rise to airway obstruction a tracheostomy is sometimes necessary.

801   The first step is an attempt to make a diagnosis on the basis of the history and physical examination. With a

lipoma or sebaceous cyst, this may be all that is
necessary before proceeding to surgical removal if
indicated. A lump apparently arising in the thyroid
gland may require thyroid function tests or a scan
before deciding on treatment. A problem arises when
the lump has no special diagnostic features and when
appropriate blood tests and x-rays have not helped
with the diagnosis. A malignant lymph node is often
suspected, in which case a thorough examination of the
upper air and food passages should precede open
biopsy.

802   The two main indications for tracheostomy are to allow
prolonged artificial ventilation and to relieve airway
obstruction. The former applies in major trauma and
postoperative chest complications; if a peroral
endotracheal tube cannot be removed after 10 to 14
days, tracheostomy is required to allow continued
adequate tracheal suction and to reduce the dead
space. Causes of acute airway obstruction include
trauma to the head and neck as a result of traffic
accidents, oedema due to allergy or infection, and
carcinoma of the larynx.

803   Close nursing observation and supervision is essential
at all times during the first 24 hours after a
tracheostomy. This entails the provision of a special
nurse or at least moving the patient to a bed adjacent
to the nursing station. Humidification should be
continuous for at least the first three days and suction
should be carried out as often as necessary, but every
hour at least. Without these precautions secretions
become thick and viscous, and dry to form crusts which
obstruct the airway. Physiotherapy is necessary to
help clear the chest since coughing is difficult when the
larynx is bypassed. In addition, a sterile technique for
dressings and the routine taking of swabs and sputum
cultures will help identify any infections. The first tube
change is done at around three to five days in the
presence of a doctor.

The eye

804   There is either unilateral or bilateral proptosis
associated with lid retraction and lid lag. Incomplete
lid closure (lagophthalmos) may result in corneal
drying due to interference with the blink reflex.
Chronic inflammatory cell infiltration of the external
ocular muscles may cause restricted eye movements
and increased intra-orbital pressure. This in turn
results in increased venous pressure, lid oedema and

optic disc swelling. The two most serious complications which may lead to blindness are perforation of the eye due to drying, and optic nerve compression.

805 I would first measure the corrected distance visual acuities in each eye before testing the pupil reactions to light. I would then examine the anterior segment for evidence of inflammation (iritis) and both fundi, if possible through a dilated pupil. During this examination I would look for evidence of retinal or vitreous haemorrhage, a retinal tear or detachment, choroiditis or neoplasia.

806 The commonest cause of unilateral proptosis in a woman of this age is dysthyroid eye disease. Other less common causes include a meningioma, haemangioma, metastatic deposits from, for example, carcinoma of the breast, or lymphoma.

807 Retrolental fibroplasia—this develops as a fibrovascular proliferation following excessive oxygenation of the immature retinal vasculature. The incidence may be reduced if the arterial Po_2 is monitored, and should be maintained below 160 mmHg.

808 Blurring of vision due to papilloedema is a common presenting symptom of a cerebral tumour causing raised intracranial pressure. Involvement of the visual pathways by a tumour may produce gradually enlarging field defects, and disorders of ocular movement may result from cranial nerve palsies. A ptosis or dilated pupil may be an early sign of a third nerve palsy, and rarely tumours may present with a specific defect of accommodation. Finally, direct orbital extension of an intracranial tumour may cause proptosis.

809 Sarcoidosis may be manifest in the external eye by the presence of multiple small conjunctival granulomata or the presence of dry eyes due to lacrimal gland involvement. Anterior uveitis (iritis) is common and may be associated with the presence of iris nodules. Posterior segment changes include posterior uveitis, retinal vasculitis and optic disc swelling due to involvement of the optic nerve.

810 In conjunctivitis the inflammation is usually accompanied by a sticky mucous discharge and the pain takes the form of a gritty, foreign-body sensation. In iritis, pain is usually more severe with intense photophobia and may be accompanied by watering and blurred vision.

811 The ocular features include blepharitis, conjunctivitis, keratitis (which may be neuroparalytic in origin) and iritis with secondary glaucoma. Transient ocular motor palsies also occur sometimes. Ocular involvement in cases of herpes zoster ophthalmicus is said to be more common where the rash involves the side of the nose indicating involvement of the nasociliary branch.

812 A chalazion is a small hard nodule found in the eyelids which arises in the Meibomian glands usually as a result of infection. Pathologically it has some of the features of a chronic granuloma, and when it persists for more than a few weeks is best treated by incision and curettage.

813 A dendritic ulcer is caused by herpes simplex virus infection of the cornea. Treatment consists of application of an antiviral ointment such as idoxuridine or acycloguanosine five times daily for up to two weeks, or until healing has occurred. Photophobia may be relieved by a mydriatic or the wearing of dark glasses. Steroid preparations should never be used as these result in enlargement of the ulcer, delayed healing, and increased scarring.

814 This includes congenital abnormalities such as blockage of the lower end of the nasolacrimal duct, congenital entropion and trichiasis, and congenital glaucoma (buphthalmos). Infective causes include ophthalmia neonatorum due to chlamydial infection.

815 The diagnosis of a corneal abrasion would first be suspected from a history of trauma and confirmed by the instillation of florescein drops, which stain a corneal epithelial defect bright green. The treatment includes a mydriatic (atropine) to relieve pain as a result of ciliary spasm, antibiotic ointment (chloramphenicol) to prevent infection, and a pad and bandage to keep the eye closed in order to encourage re-epithelialization. The eye should be inspected the following day in order to make sure that healing is occurring and that there is no infection.

816 Subconjunctival haemorrhage is most commonly idiopathic. Known causes include coughing, vascular abnormalities, and blood dyscrasias. It may also occur following trauma, and in these cases, if a posterior limit to the haemorrhage on the eyeball cannot be identified, bony injury to the orbit or anterior cranial fossa should be excluded.

817 The most important first aid measure is immediate irrigation using a cold tap or immersion in a bucket of cold water. In a casualty department the eye should be

irrigated with buffered salt solution following local anaesthetic drops (amethocaine)—then the visual acuity assessed. Subsequent management depends on the precise nature of the chemical, and if possible a sample of it should be tested with universal indicator paper in order to discover its pH. Severe burns require admission to hospital whereas minor burns (those not involving strong acid or alkali) may be treated with mydriatics and antibiotics.

818 Congenital melanin pigmentation of the conjunctiva is usually benign and of little significance. Acquired pigmentation however may indicate the development of a precancerous melanosis or a melanoma and therefore requires full investigation including biopsy.

819 An attack of acute glaucoma may start with the development of haloes (i.e., coloured rings around lights) associated with blurring of vision in one or both eyes. Later the eye may become painful and a severe headache develops. Nausea and vomiting may occur.

820 In acute glaucoma the eye becomes congested, with a vertically oval, fixed, semi-dilated pupil. The cornea is hazy and examination of the position of the iris shows a shallow anterior chamber. The eye feels hard, reflecting the increased intra-ocular pressure. The optic disc is difficult to visualize, but it may be normal or swollen during an acute attack and may not appear atrophic until several weeks after the attack.

821 Acute closed angle glaucoma usually occurs in patients with a shallow anterior chamber and an associated narrow filtration angle. When the pupils of such eyes are semi-dilated (for example in dimly lit conditions and under adrenergic stimulation) the iris root may come into contact with the posterior peripheral cornea thus preventing aqueous outflow through the filtration angle.

822 Chronic simple glaucoma has an insidious onset and in its early stages the patient is usually asymptomatic. Later the patient may become aware of progressive defects in his visual field but these may not be noticed until the patient has tunnel vision as a result of gross peripheral field loss. Visual acuity is not reduced until a very advanced stage when the central fixation is affected. The cardinal sign of chronic simple glaucoma is the development of a pathologically cupped optic disc which is always associated with field defects.

823 Keratic precipitates are clumps of leucocytes which are adherent to the corneal endothelium and are seen as small white dots in cases of iritis.

824 Drugs may lower intra-ocular pressure by reducing aqueous secretion, promoting aqueous outflow or as osmotic agents. Acetazolamide is a carbonic anhydrase inhibitor which reduces aqueous secretion. Pilocarpine acts by constricting the pupil and pulling the iris root away from the trabecular meshwork, thus restoring the outflow facility to the eye. Intravenous mannitol or oral glycerol are examples of osmotic agents.

825 An intra-ocular foreign body should always be suspected where there is a history of metal striking metal at the time of an eye injury. The eye may look relatively normal if there is a small entry wound but the diagnosis is usually evident on examination of the pupil. A poorly reacting pupil suggests loss of the anterior chamber due to leakage of aqueous, while distortion of the pupil margin indicates iris prolapse or iridodialysis. If the fundal view through the pupil is obscured this may be due either to the presence of blood or to lens opacities. X-ray of the orbit should always be taken whenever the diagnosis is suspected.

826 Congenital cataracts may be associated with maternal infections such as rubella, cytomegalovirus and toxoplasmosis. Other causes in children include Down's syndrome, Turner's syndrome, galactosaemia, Still's disease and severe atopic disease. In adults the commonest condition associated with cataracts is diabetes mellitus but other less common associations include hypoparathyroidism and dystrophia myotonica. Steroids and chlorpromazine are examples of drugs which may induce cataract formation.

827 Aphakia is absence of the lens. The optical correction of an eye following lens removal requires a thick convex glass which magnifies the image by approximately one-third. Other disadvantages include image distortion due to spherical aberration and a ring scotoma whilst using the spectacles. If only one eye is aphakic double vision prevents the use of both eyes together unless a contact lens is used.

828 Surgery may be indicated when bilateral cataracts prevent the patient from continuing normal activities; this usually occurs when the fully corrected visual acuity in the better eye falls to approximately 6/18. A uni-ocular cataract may sometimes be removed in order to prevent the complications of a mature lens or if binocular vision is needed and the patient is willing and able to tolerate a contact or intra-ocular lens.

829 The patient usually complains of discomfort behind the eye which is more marked on movement of the eye. The patient notices the development of a central scotoma

which may enlarge within hours, or more usually days, to produce profound visual loss and fixation is affected.

830 There is loss of the direct pupil reflex in the left eye with preservation of the consensual left response (when light is shone on the right eye).

831 There is a pinkish discolouration of the disc associated with engorgement of veins and loss of spontaneous venous pulsation. Later the disc margins become blurred and the nerve fibres swell to produce elevation of the disc. Gross papilloedema is associated with haemorrhages in the nerve fibre layer in and around the disc.

832 There are two main clinical types—background and proliferative retinopathy. Background retinopathy consists of the presence of micro-aneurysms, beading of veins, small blot haemorrhages and hard exudates. This form of retinopathy is associated with visual loss due to macular oedema or retinal capillary closure. Proliferative retinopathy is characterized by the formation of new vessels either in or on the retina or arising from the optic disc. Visual loss occurs as a result of haemorrhage into the vitreous or the development of fibrosis leading to secondary retinal detachment.

833 Yes. In background retinopathy, laser photocoagulation can be used to reduce macular oedema by coagulating leaking blood vessels. Early proliferative retinopathy is also treated with a laser but in advanced cases with retinal detachment the only treatment is surgical and the results are frequently unsuccessful.

834 The patient may complain of blurred or distorted vision if the choroid near the macula is involved. A small focus of choroiditis may not produce any symptoms, but floaters may develop due to the presence of inflammatory cells in the vitreous.

835 Choroidal melanoma commonly presents without symptoms as a pigmented lesion discovered on routine ophthalmoscopy. More advanced cases may present with secondary retinal detachment or secondary glaucoma. Distant metastatic disease (for example an enlarged liver), is a rare but well recognized form of presentation.

836 Night blindness is a defect in dark adaptation associated with abnormal function of retinal rods. It may be a congenital disorder, not associated with any obvious fundus change, or it may be a presenting feature of inherited retinitis pigmentosa when the

fundal changes include pigment clumping with narrowing of the retinal arteries and optic atrophy. The commonest cause of acquired night blindness is vitamin A deficiency when it may also be associated with keratomalacia.

837   Causes of sudden visual loss include retinal artery occlusion due to either embolism or thrombosis, central retinal vein or branch vein occlusion, vitreous haemorrhage, retinal detachment, optic neuritis, and toxic optic neuropathy due to methyl alcohol poisoning.

838   Amblyopia is a condition of diminished vision which is not associated with any structural abnormality of the afferent visual pathways.

839   Pupil constriction occurs with parasympathetic stimulation either directly with acetylcholine and pilocarpine or indirectly with drugs which prevent the breakdown of acetylcholine such as physostigmine and phospholine iodide. Pupil dilatation is brought about either by sympathomimetic agents including adrenaline and phenylephrine or parasympathetic antagonists which include atropine, homatropine, hyosine and cyclopentolate.

840   There are three indications for squint surgery—to restore binocular single vision, to correct an abnormal head posture due to ocular torticollis and to produce a satisfactory cosmetic appearance.

841   This is an early sign of chiasmal compression which is usually due to a pituitary adenoma. Other pathology in the same region may produce similar field changes and the differential diagnosis includes a cranio-pharyngioma, suprasellar meningioma, and an aneurysm of the anterior communicating artery.

842   The differential diagnosis of a white pupil in childhood includes a congenital cataract, retinoblastoma, retrolental fibroplasia, choroiditis, retinal colobomata, and persistent primary hyperplastic vitreous.

Orthopaedics and fractures

Fractures: general

843   The difference is that a compound fracture communicates with the exterior through a defect in the skin, while a simple or 'closed' fracture does not. The importance lies in the danger of infection which is much greater in a compound fracture.

844 A pathological fracture is a fracture through bone which is abnormal for one reason or another. There are a large number of conditions which may weaken the bone, but a good example would be a secondary malignant deposit. Other common causes for pathological fractures are benign bone tumours (such as enchondroma) and Paget's disease.

845 The best known stress fracture is the 'march' fracture which occurs in a metatarsal bone. It was described in army recruits on route marches, hence the name of the fracture. Other bones, almost always weight-bearing, may develop stress fracture.

846 This is a common surgical emergency. The danger lies in the possibility that soft tissue or bony infection will occur. The patient should be given antibiotics and tetanus prophylaxis and then taken to theatre within six hours of injury. The wound should be surgically cleaned with removal of all contaminated or non-viable tissue, and in all but the most minor compound injuries the wound should be left unsutured. The fracture can be treated in various ways such as skeletal traction, internal or external fixation or plaster but, whichever is chosen, it should not interfere with dressing the soft tissue injury.

847 The principal danger is that swelling inside the rigid plaster will impair circulation to the distal part of the limb, resulting in gangrene. The danger can be avoided either by splitting the plaster until you can see the skin, or by initially applying a backslab and completing the plaster later.

848 Skeletal traction is a method of holding a fracture reduced by the application of traction via a pin placed through a more distal bone. The commonest example is the femoral shaft fracture treated using a pin through the upper tibia. Another application is in the treatment of tibial and ankle fractures using a calcaneal pin.

849 Fracture disease was described by the German surgeon Bohler and consists of all the secondary changes that occur in a fractured limb that has been immobilized for a long time. These changes include wasting of the muscle, osteoporosis of the bone, and stiffness of the joints. Sometimes these changes can be very incapacitating and the patient will hardly use the affected limb at all.

850 Callus is a mass of immature bone which forms as part of the healing process of a fracture. It forms a cuff around the broken bone ends and helps stabilize the fracture while union progresses. The callus is

gradually remodelled to form mature bone but this
process may take months if not years.

851   Patients with major closed fractures may die of blood
       loss which can easily be underestimated. One and a
       half litres of blood can be lost into the soft tissues
       around a fractured femur. (With pelvic fractures blood
       loss is even greater.) It is very important, therefore,
       that resuscitation is started as soon as possible. Blood
       should be cross-matched urgently and a careful eye
       should be kept upon the pulse, blood pressure, urinary
       output and central venous pressure.

852   Fat embolism usually occurs two to three days after
       fracture of a major bone. The patient becomes restless,
       confused, sometimes aggressive and then lapses into
       unconsciousness. Petechial haemorrhages occur over
       the upper half of the body in 50 per cent of cases. The
       arterial blood gases must be measured and the Po_2 will
       often be found to be less than half the normal
       100 mmHg.

853   The causes include excessive movement at the fracture
       site, distraction of the fracture, muscle interposition,
       sepsis, poor blood supply, synovial fluid in the fracture
       line, pre-existing bone pathology, advanced age, poor
       nutrition and steroid therapy.

854   Volkmann's contracture is fibrosis and shortening of
       muscles due to ischaemia. Classically this affects the
       long flexor muscles of the forearm giving rise to a claw
       hand so that the fingers can only be extended when the
       wrist is flexed. Very often there is accompanying nerve
       damage so that there are also sensory changes. The
       commonest cause is a supracondylar fracture of the
       humerus which injures the brachial artery.

855   Nerve damage is divided according to its severity into
       three grades: neuropraxia, axonotmesis and
       neurotmesis. In neuropraxia conduction is interrupted
       for a short time only and will return fully in a matter of
       hours. Axonotmesis implies sufficient damage for
       axons to degenerate distal to the injury; however, the
       nerve is not completely disrupted and regeneration can
       be expected. In neurotmesis the nerve is completely
       disrupted and reinnervation will not occur without
       surgical repair. In practice these grades may co-exist
       in the same nerve, and give uneven recovery.

856   Regeneration of nerves proceeds at the rate of about an
       inch a month, so that more proximal injuries take
       longer to recover. Another month must be allowed for
       reinnervation of motor end-plates. The first evidence of
       recovery is usually seen on EMG with clinical
       improvement several weeks later. After about 18

months of denervation the motor end-plates will not recover so that motor reinnervation is not possible.

Orthopaedics: general

857 *Staph. aureus* is responsible in 80 per cent of cases. It reaches the bone via the blood, usually from a septic focus elsewhere. The infection tends to lodge in the metaphyseal region of the bone where blood supply is greatest.

858 The child is ill, pyrexial, anorexic, restless but not moving the affected limb which will probably be red, swollen, warm and is painful, particularly if moved. The white cell count and ESR are raised. The diagnosis can be particularly difficult to make in babies and should be borne in mind in the infant who is unwell with no obvious cause.

859 Acute osteomyelitis should be treated early and vigorously if complete resolution is to be achieved. If chronic osteomyelitis is allowed to supervene then cure is extremely difficult to achieve. Blood cultures should be taken to try to identify the organism and then high doses of bactericidal antibiotics should be given. Fucidic acid with flucloxicillin is a popular combination therapy. The place of surgery is not completely agreed upon but drainage should be performed if subperiosteal pus is thought to be present.

860 Dead bone, infected granulation tissue and pus within the bone, all part of chronic osteomyelitis, allow organisms to flourish, especially as penetration by antibiotics is poor in this condition.

861 Metal or cement predispose to bony infection and make eradication of infection more difficult. If an implant is inserted into a bone which has been infected in the past there is a considerable risk of making the infection active again.

862 The risk is about one to two per cent of developing deep infection. To keep the rate as low as possible all septic foci should be treated before surgery. Prophylactic antibiotics have been shown to be effective and meticulous attention to sterility in the operating theatre is very important.

863 Rheumatoid arthritis, particularly when treated with steroids, presents some special hazards in surgery. Resistance to infection is lower, which is of particular importance when considering joint replacement. The bone is osteoporotic and will not hold surgical implants as well as normal bones. The skin is often thin and there may be a vasculitis leading to wound necrosis.

Finally, it is important to x-ray the neck before embarking upon anaesthesia as there may well be a potentially unstable lesion in the cervical spine.

864 Almost any tissue can be damaged. The articular cartilage is attacked early in the disease leading to loss of joint space, the adjacent bone may be eroded, joint capsule and ligaments may become soft and degenerate, while tendons may be weakened and eventually rupture.

865 The commonest deformity is an ulnar deviation at the MCP joints and it is very often accompanied by volar subluxation or dislocation of the proximal phalanges on the metacarpal heads. The joints may well be swollen due to the synovitis. The mechanism of ulnar drift is not certain but once it has begun the long flexor and extensor tendons tend to increase the deformity.

866 Ankylosing spondylitis most commonly affects young adult males. The spine and the costovertebral joints are most commonly affected leading to stiffness of the spine and poor chest expansion. Later on, the spine may ankylose in a kyphotic position leading to an ugly deformity. The large joints, particularly the hips and knees may also become progressively more stiff. Maintenance of the range of movement and the use of anti-inflammatory drugs are the mainstay of treatment but surgery can be useful. Joint replacement is often very successful in these patients and in certain circumstances spinal osteotomy may make a tremendous difference to a severe kyphosis.

867 Osteoporosis is the loss of bone substance, including osteoid tissue, while osteomalacia is the demineralization of bone without loss of osteoid. Osteomalacia in children is known as rickets. The blood chemistry is usually normal in osteoporosis whereas in osteomalacia there is a high serum alkaline phosphatase and probably a high urinary calcium.

868 Osteoporosis is a very common condition and is always present to some degree in postmenopausal females, making them more prone to fractures. Disuse of the limb, due perhaps to immobilization in plaster, will cause osteoporosis while the whole skeleton will be affected if a patient is confined to bed for a few weeks. Osteoporosis is an accepted consequence of weightlessness experienced on a space flight. Rheumatoid arthritis and the steroids that are commonly used to treat the condition are both causes of osteoporosis.

869 Paget's disease of bone is a disorder of the normally continuous remodelling process. It may be due to a

virus but the aetiology is unclear. It is a very common
condition whose incidence increases with age,
although it is usually asymptomatic. It causes the
bones to become thicker and to lose their normal
internal architecture, so that although they look
widened and sclerotic on x-ray, there is often bowing of
long bones and pathological fractures may occur. When
pain occurs it may be due to fissure fractures in the
bowed and weakened bone. Secondary osteo-arthritis
may occur in adjacent joints. Two rare complications
are high output cardiac failure due to bony arterial
shunts and osteosarcoma which is rapidly fatal.

870   An achondroplastic dwarf has short limbs while the
      trunk and skull are relatively normal. This is due to a
      defect in the formation of bones which ossify from
      cartilage. Achondroplasiacs have normal intelligence
      and good musculature and are often employed as circus
      dwarfs. They are at risk of developing spinal stenosis
      and hydrocephalus but the condition is compatible
      with a normal life span.

871   Severe haemophiliacs are likely to get recurrent
      haemarthrosis of the major joints after little or no
      trauma; this can lead to severe secondary changes in
      the joints with fixed deformities. Such damage can be
      minimized by prompt splinting of the joint and
      treatment with factor VIII. Permanent damage to
      peripheral nerves can be caused by pressure from
      expanding haematomas and prompt measures are
      needed to prevent this.

872   Secondary deposits are far more common than primary
      bone tumours. Almost any tumour may spread to bone
      but there are five that classically do so—carcinoma of
      the breast, bronchus, kidney, thyroid, and prostate.
      Simple clinical examination and investigation of these
      organs will often save the patient an unnecessary bone
      biopsy.

873   Osteosarcoma occurs most commonly in males between
      the ages of 10 and 30. The common sites, in order of
      frequency, are the lower end of the femur, upper tibia,
      upper humerus, distal radius and proximal femur.
      There are only 150 new cases of osteosarcoma a year in
      England and Wales and to detect such a tumour it is
      important to have an index of suspicion. Rarely,
      osteosarcoma is secondary to radiation therapy or
      Paget's disease.

874   The treatment advocated by Sir Stanford Cade was
      initial radiotherapy of the tumour and to delay
      amputation until six months had elapsed without
      evidence of pulmonary metastases. The idea behind

this treatment was to save the large proportion who were going to die from having an unnecessary amputation. This method has been superseded by immediate amputation and high-dose chemotherapy. It is hoped that the chemotherapy can deal with micrometastases in the lung, and so far it seems that this method gives an improved long-term survival.

875 Osteotomy is surgical division and refixation of a bone. It may be used to correct deformities such as bow leg; to reposition part of a joint, for example, the head of the femur in congenital dislocation of the hip; or for its non-specific pain relieving effect when a bone is divided near a joint.

876 Hemiarthroplasty is the reshaping or replacement of one half of a joint. The most common application is replacement of the head of the femur following subcapital femoral neck fracture in the elderly.

877 Débridement is the surgical cleaning of a wound including excision of all grossly contaminated, dead and doubtfully viable tissue. It is particularly important that dead muscle is carefully excised as it is a perfect culture medium for anaerobic bacilli.

878 The commonly used metals are stainless steel, chrome cobalt alloy, and titanium. A convex metal surface usually articulates with a concave surface of high density polyethylene. The other material in wide use is silastic, for the replacement of small joints such as in fingers and toes.

879 The most common cause is infection which occurs in about one per cent of cases. Late failure may occur due to aseptic loosening of components.

Orthopaedics: regional

The hip and femur

880 True leg length is measured from the anterior superior iliac spine to the medial malleolus, while apparent length is measured from the umbilicus or xiphisternum to the medial malleolus. While true shortening indicates abnormality within the leg, apparent shortening is simply due to tilting of the pelvis. The most common cause of this tilting is a fixed adduction deformity at one hip which forces the patient to tilt the pelvis to avoid having to walk with his legs crossed.

881 The Trendelenburg test is a test of the integrity of the abductor mechanism of the hip and is performed by

asking the patient to stand on one leg. The test is positive if the opposite side of the pelvis drops down below the horizontal. The commonest cause of a positive test is pain due to arthritis in the hip, but it may also be positive if the abductor muscles themselves are weak or if the pivot around which they act is not functioning, for example after excision of the head of the femur.

882 Fixed flexion deformity of the hip is measured by the use of Thomas's test. In this test the patient lies on his back and any lumbar lordosis and pelvic tilting are eliminated by flexing the opposite hip as far as possible—a hand can be placed under the small of the patient's back to make sure the back is touching the couch. If the thigh comes off the couch there is fixed flexion deformity which is measured as the angle between the thigh and the horizontal.

883 The blood supply to the head of the femur runs in the capsule applied to the neck of the femur with little if any supply via the ligamentum teres. The vascularity of the head is therefore endangered if the capsule is stretched or disrupted. This may occur with fracture of the neck of the femur, dislocation of the hip joint or the maintenance of an extreme position of the hip joint as may occur during treatment for congenital dislocation of the hip.

884 The bony contours of the ball and socket articulation provide considerable stability, enhanced by the fibrocartilaginous labrum around the edge of the acetabulum which deepens it. The thick joint capsule, condensed to form the iliofemoral, pubofemoral and ischiofemoral ligaments, and the muscles which cross the hip joint add to the stability. Considerable force is required to dislocate this joint.

885 Typically this fracture produces a shortened, externally rotated, painful leg. In the elderly, who are particularly susceptible to this fracture, and in the demented, pain may not be severe and inability to walk may be more important as a clinical feature. If the fracture is impacted, the classical deformity will not be present and the patient, although complaining of pain, may be able to walk. Therefore an x-ray is necessary in the elderly patient complaining of hip pain. The mortality approaches 30 per cent by three months, primarily due to the loss of mobility in an elderly patient leading to pneumonia, bed sores, urinary infection, deep vein thrombosis, etc.

886 Replacement of the femoral head following *intracapsular* fracture is the usual treatment because

the alternative, reduction and pinning, has drawbacks in this injury. These include the likelihood of non-union of the fracture, avascular necrosis of the head of the femur, and cutting out of the pin from osteoporotic bone on attempted weight bearing. Replacement of the head of the femur, although a more major procedure, allows early return to full mobility, so vital in the elderly patient.

887 Posterior dislocation of the hip requires considerable violence and may therefore be associated with other severe injuries which may distract attention from the hip. The most likely decoy is an ipsilateral fracture of the femoral shaft which will account for pain in the region and will disguise the characteristic fixed adducted posture which the dislocated hip will assume. Posterior dislocation of the hip joint should not be missed if a careful examination of the patient is undertaken.

888 Central dislocation of the hip is really a fracture-dislocation in which the head of the femur is forced through the acetabulum into the pelvis. The head of the femur is itself quite likely to have received considerable damage. Reconstruction is very difficult and a good result unlikely.

889 This condition should be diagnosed as soon after birth as possible as treatment is then easier and more effective. It is a clinical diagnosis, reached during routine examination of the infant. The main clinical signs are loss of abduction and a clunk or click of reduction which occurs when the hip is placed in the stable position of flexion and abduction. Asymmetry of skin creases may be seen around the hip joint in a unilateral dislocation but this is an unreliable sign. Later on there is development of a fixed flexion deformity and further limitation of abduction. Radiology is not of much help until the proximal femoral epiphysis begins to ossify at the age of three or four months.

890 If congenital dislocation of the hip is treated early it is usually quite easy to obtain a sound reduction, and from there development of the hip proceeds normally. On the other hand, if the dislocation is not discovered until the child has learned to walk, a number of secondary deformities are likely to have developed, making treatment considerably more difficult—open reduction of the dislocation may then be required and osteotomies of the femur and pelvis may be needed to obtain a stable hip.

891 The condition is commoner in females by a factor of six. The other risk factors are breech presentation, first-born babies, oligohydramnios, Caucasian race and

positive family history. It is important to know the epidemiological facts about CDH so that those at risk may be carefully watched.

892 The pathological process in Perthes' disease is one of recurrent episodes of avascular necrosis of the whole or part of the femoral capital epiphysis, the cause of which has not been established. If the degree of necrosis is minor, then replacement of the dead bone occurs without permanent disability, while if a large amount of the head is affected, collapse of the femoral head will occur with varying degrees of flattening when healing finally occurs.

893 It is important first to decide whether any treatment is necessary—in those with minor degrees of involvement the spherical shape of the femoral head is not endangered and healing will occur without treatment. In more severe cases, treatment is aimed at containing the head within the acetabulum; in this way it is hoped that the softened bone will be moulded by the acetabulum, producing a congruous hip. Containment may be achieved either by a rather inconvenient splint or by femoral osteotomy. Some advocate non-weight-bearing until regeneration has occurred but this may take months or years and can be very trying for the growing child.

894 A mild or moderate pain in the groin or knee may be the only symptom. The patient, usually a young adolescent, may develop a slight limp and later a deformity consisting of shortening and external rotation of the affected leg. This is a deceptive condition and may be difficult to diagnose.

895 A lateral x-ray of the hip is needed because the slip tends to occur in a posterior direction and may be missed in the early stages if only an AP film is taken. Adequate hip x-rays may not be ordered if the patient's pain is mainly in the knee.

896 Total hip replacement has such wide indications that the alternatives may be neglected. Foremost among these is upper femoral osteotomy which will often give years of pain relief and avoids total joint replacement in a younger patient. Arthrodesis may be satisfactory for a young man, likely to make heavy demands on his hip and is also indicated when old osteomyelitis makes total joint replacement risky. Other operations, such as Girdlestone excision arthroplasty and hemi-arthroplasty are rarely used these days.

897 The presence of sepsis elsewhere in the body is an important contra-indication which must be dealt with before operation is performed. Old sepsis around the

affected joint is also a considerable danger. Loss of bone stock for any reason means that it is very difficult to fix the components of the hip joint securely to the bone. Youth is a relative contra-indication to total hip replacement as revision operations are more likely to be required in the younger and more vigorous patient.

898 An acute septic arthritis of the hip should not be difficult to diagnose except in a very young child unable to indicate the site of pain. The hip is stiff and painful to move and there is a severe systemic upset with pyrexia and a raised white cell count and sedimentation rate. Less acute infection may be more difficult to identify particularly in a deep joint such as the hip. In such cases aspiration of the hip, as well as the usual blood cultures, may be necessary to establish the diagnosis.

899 In the early stages there is loss of joint space due to erosion of the articular cartilage. Erosions around the edges of the articular surfaces are likely to occur and there may well be a generalized loss of bone density. As time goes on, secondary changes typical of osteo-arthritis may be imposed upon the original rheumatoid changes.

900 The femur should be splinted, an intravenous infusion started, blood taken for cross-matching, and analgesia given. Splintage, usually with a Thomas's splint, will minimize further damage to soft tissues, reduce bleeding into the thigh and lessen pain. Volume replacement should be started early as blood loss into the thigh may be up to 2 litres. Analgesia should be given before all the painful steps associated with radiological examination, provided there are no contra-indications such as head injury. Small intravenous doses of opiate are preferable to intramuscular injections which may be absorbed very slowly in such circumstances. In short, emergency treatment aims to stabilize the general condition prior to definitive treatment of the fracture.

901 It consists of a leather covered ring around the root of the limb and a metal loop running down the length of the limb. The leg is rested on slings between the two sides of the metal loop and traction can be applied over the end of the loop providing very effective splintage. Various adaptations can be made to this basic arrangement—for example, the limb can be plastered into the splint, producing the so-called Tobruk plaster which permits pain-free transport. Thomas's splint is a simple piece of apparatus which has made an immense difference to the mortality from fractures of the femur.

The knee and lower leg

902 The menisci perform two useful functions—they act to spread a considerable proportion of the load across the knee joint so that point loading does not occur, and they have a role in spreading synovial fluid around the joint and thus nourishing the articular cartilage. The menisci used to be thought to have little if any use, so that their removal would do little damage. However, it has now been shown that their removal causes considerable damage to the joint and is likely to lead to osteo-arthritis of the knee.

903 In adults there is a physiological valgus of about 7 degrees between femur and tibia. There is a range of normality between about 2 degrees and 11 degrees with women tending towards the higher values. In children these angles do not apply as very small children often develop bow legs followed by knock knees and end up perfectly normal adults. The physiological valgus must be taken into account in total knee replacement.

904 A 'locked' knee has a block to full extension, usually as a result of trauma. This may be quite a subtle sign, with only the last few degrees of normal hyperextension missing from the range. Sometimes intermittent locking will occur, when the patient finds the knee will not straighten past a certain point; however, if he manipulates the knee, suddenly the full range of movement returns. The usual causes of a locked knee are a torn meniscus or a loose body in the knee.

905 Lateral or medial strain should be applied to the knee in about 20 degrees of flexion, as the anatomy of the knee is such that it is stable to such strains when fully extended, even if the collateral ligaments are divided. It is important to test the other knee as the degree of normal laxity varies considerably from person to person. Isolated collateral ligament damage is rare—the cruciate ligaments and possibly other structures may have been injured as well.

906 If the knee is damaged for any reason there is rapid wasting of the quadriceps muscle. The vastus medialis is the component that shows this wasting first and is usually the last to recover. Other muscles in the limb will undergo wasting but the quadriceps is particularly important as it contributes to the strength and stability of the knee. Rehabilitation programmes for the knee are designed primarily to rebuild quadriceps power.

907 The site of tenderness can be useful in determining the nature of the injury. If there is collateral ligament damage it usually occurs close to the origin or insertion of the ligament and so tenderness is away from the joint

line. If the tenderness is at the joint line, the diagnosis
is likely to be capsular or meniscal damage.

908 Stressed films of the knee in valgus or varus strain
may be useful in showing an increased joint space on
one side which indicates a tear of the collateral
ligaments. Arthrography with contrast alone or
contrast with air can be useful, particularly to show
damage to the menisci. Arthroscopy is becoming more
commonly used, enabling accurate diagnosis of most
intra-articular pathology though it requires
anaesthesia and admission to hospital.

909 Tears most commonly begin in the posterior region of
the medial meniscus. This area of the meniscus can be
caught between the femur and tibia by a sudden twist
on the flexed knee. Once the tear has begun it is likely
to extend round to the front of the meniscus and may
eventually produce a complete 'bucket handle' tear.

910 It used to be thought that removal of the meniscus was
a harmless procedure, but on long-term follow up it has
been shown that osteo-arthritis of the knee is a
common consequence which may occur many years
later. It has also become apparent from autopsy studies
that asymptomatic meniscal tears are common; for this
reason surgeons are becoming more conservative in
their indications for meniscectomy.

911 This differential diagnosis is difficult because severe
pain prevents adequate testing for instability, so it
may be necessary to examine the knee under local or
general anaesthesia. Stressed radiographs may also
help. It is important to distinguish partial from
complete tears which often benefit from early surgical
repair.

912 This is a condition in which there is gradual separation
of an osteochondral fragment from a surface within the
knee joint. The commonest site is on the lateral side of
the medial femoral condyle. It often occurs in athletic
teenagers and young adults, causing pain and swelling
with occasional locking or giving way particularly if
the fragment becomes completely separated.

913 Unstable patella is a term which describes a range of
conditions. In its mildest form this can be a slight
abnormality of tracking of the patella in the
intercondylar groove leading to retropatellar pain. At
the opposite end of the scale is congenital dislocation of
the patella when the patella lies lateral to the knee
joint. Between these extremes the patella may
subluxate or dislocate with varying degrees of
readiness. The mildest degrees of instability may be
helped by physiotherapy aimed at increasing muscle

control of the patella but in more marked instability some form of surgical realignment of the patella is required.

914 Genu varum is bow legs. In this condition the weight of the body is taken mainly or entirely through the medial compartment of the knee joint, leading to loss of articular cartilage. In advanced cases there may be bony collapse of the medial tibial plateau or the medial femoral condyle which will make the deformity worse. Pain is caused by the degenerative arthritis on the medial side of the joint and possibly also by traction on the lateral ligamentous structures.

915 The alternative operations for severe rheumatoid arthritis of the knee are osteotomy, arthrodesis, and total knee replacement. Osteotomy will give relief of pain provided the destruction of the joint surfaces is not severe. In advanced cases the choice is between arthrodesis, which will give a stiff but pain free knee, and a knee replacement, which should give a mobile, pain free knee. Unfortunately knee replacement cannot be relied upon to last for more than five years. All these factors must be weighed up before a particular operative treatment is suggested. Synovectomy of the knee can be useful in relatively early rheumatoid arthritis but cannot help when severe destruction has already occurred.

916 A displaced fracture needs accurate repair or possibly excision of the patella and repair of the expansion, after which the knee is splinted for some weeks. If a fracture is undisplaced, the extensor mechanism remains intact, so that splintage is necessary only for a short period.

917 In Osgood-Schlatter's disease the patellar tendon pulls on the apophysis of the tibial tubercle and produces gradual avulsion with new bone formation. This is due to disproportion between the strength of the quadriceps and the hardness of the bone. As the apophysis closes the symptoms will resolve.

918 The standard method of treating a closed fracture of the tibial shaft is to manipulate it into a satisfactory position which is then held in an above-knee plaster until union of the fracture has occurred. Newer treatments include internal fixation and functional bracing, but treatment in plaster is very successful if carefully applied, and the newer methods must be measured against it.

919 External fixation is an arrangement whereby a fractured bone is held steady by a system of external scaffolding. The bone is held by two or three pins above

and below the fracture site, connected by means of adjustable clamps. The advantages are that a compound fracture can be stabilized without metal in the wound, and that the wound can be dressed or skin grafted without disturbing the splint.

The ankle and foot

920 Sprained ankle is usually an inversion injury with damage to the lateral ligament of the ankle joint, the anterior and middle components of this ligament usually receiving the brunt of the damage. In the majority of cases there is only a partial tear and full recovery occurs, but if there is a complete tear of one or more of the components of the lateral ligament there may be a permanent disability.

921 In ankle fractures the final functional result is closely correlated with the accuracy of reduction. Large forces pass through this complex joint which has a relatively small surface area so that any small malalignment or roughness of the surfaces leads to wear of the articular cartilage.

922 A bunion is a bony exostosis, often covered by a bursa, which produces a bump on the medial aspect of the head of the first metatarsal bone. Hallux valgus means angulation of the big toe in a lateral direction, leaving the head of the first metatarsal more obvious than usual. A bunion often accompanies hallux valgus, making the symptoms worse.

923 Hallux rigidus is osteo-arthritis of the first metatarsophalangeal joint. There is gradual onset of stiffness and pain and the formation of bony osteophytes around the joint, particularly on the dorsal aspect. The condition may follow old trauma or unusual strains such as occur in sporting or dancing activities.

924 Metatarsalgia is pain in the forefoot due to excessive weight bearing on one or more of the metatarsal heads, in turn producing a callosity under the foot which makes the painful area more prominent. There are several causes including toe deformities, such as claw toe; previous surgery for hallux valgus, which may stop the big toe functioning as a weight-bearing organ; fixed plantar flexion at the ankle; and loss of soft tissue padding from the sole of the foot, as may occur in rheumatoid arthritis.

925 The other name for club-foot is talipes equino varus. This term provides a description of the deformity— 'equinus' refers to plantar flexion of the foot and ankle as occurs naturally in the horse (equus),

and varus refers to inversion of the foot. In severe club foot there is a tight tendo Achillis and a high, small, inverted heel and some adduction of the forefoot. The calf and foot are smaller than normal, this becoming more noticeable as the patient gets older and persisting even if a good correction of the deformity has been achieved.

926 Flat feet are common in the young and do not cause symptoms in this age group. Later in life, as muscles and ligaments weaken, there may be further collapse of the longitudinal arch and symptoms may develop. Some flat feet may have a marked valgus deformity which may be painful. The most troublesome form of flat foot, requiring early treatment, is the rocker-bottomed foot, due to a congenitally vertical talus—in this condition the sole is actually convex and the position of the talus can be seen on x-ray.

The spine

927 If the sacral nerve roots are damaged by a central disc prolapse there will be loss of bladder function, and sometimes impotence and loss of ejaculation. Recovery may take a long time even after the compressive force has been removed, so early surgical relief is indicated.

928 The thoracic spine is less mobile than the lumbar and cervical spines and is splinted by the rib cage. Forces falling on the thoracic spine are likely to be transmitted to the more mobile segments of the spine. The cervical spine is more commonly injured nowadays, mainly in road accidents.

929 An intervertebral disc consists of an outer layer of concentric rings of tough fibrous tissue known as the annulus fibrosus, and a semi-fluid interior called the nucleus pulposus. The fibres of the annulus lie at 45 degrees to the vertebrae, and alternate layers are at right angles to each other. The nucleus pulposus, the remnant of embryonic notochord, is situated towards the posterior part of the disc. This structure allows mobility as well as efficient shock absorption.

930 Structural scoliosis, that is, a fixed rotation of the vertebrae, can best be seen if the suspected area is viewed in profile and is accentuated when the patient bends forward, when the ribs will emphasize the deformity. Another clue may be given by a high shoulder or prominent hip.

931 Limitation of straight leg raising by pain indicates tethering of the lower lumbar nerve roots, usually due to a prolapsed intervertebral disc. A useful confirmatory sign of this pathology is the sciatic

stretch test, in which the leg is raised to the level that pain permits and the foot then passively dorsiflexed—this will cause pain due to further traction on the nerve roots. Both legs may have limited straight leg raising due to tight hamstrings but this is not painful.

932 A patient with spondylolisthesis of significant degree has a shortened lumbar region with a fold in each flank and a loss of normal lordotic curve. A step may be palpable in the lumbar spine.

933 This means that the tough interspinous ligament has been disrupted and there is likely to be an unstable fracture-dislocation at this level of the spine. This sign is valuable in the fresh injury but as swelling and bruising supervene the soft area becomes less obvious.

934 A psoas abscess will point in the groin as it tracks down the psoas tendon. The other important sign is hip flexion due to psoas spasm.

935 A myelogram is performed by injecting contrast medium through a lumbar puncture needle into the spinal canal. Suitable positioning of the patient allows the cord, nerve roots and any displaced disc to be outlined.

936 This is the view used to show spondylolysis. In an oblique radiograph the pars interarticularis is thrown into prominence and a break becomes very noticeable. The posterior elements of each vertebra look rather like a 'Scottie' dog and a collar on the dog's neck is the sign of a spondylolysis.

937 In the lower cervical spine. This area, which is prone to injury, is often poorly shown on x-ray due to lack of co-operation in a patient who may be drunk or concussed. By pulling down on the arms or by taking oblique views it is possible to show this area in sufficient detail to exclude injury.

938 The vast majority of prolapsed intervertebral discs will resolve with conservative management. The patient should be rested in bed with adequate nursing and analgesia until symptoms have subsided. He can then be mobilized slowly and advised on the avoidance of back pain. Some patients will benefit from physiotherapy and weight loss. Only a small percentage of disc prolapses require surgery.

939 A disc that prolapses in a directly posterior direction, so that the sacral nerve roots are damaged bilaterally, is an urgent matter requiring early treatment. Interference with bladder function is a sign that this

has occurred and early decompression is necessary. If decompression is delayed there may be permanent urinary incontinence.

940 The term 'laminectomy' is often used loosely to mean the same as 'disc excision'. Laminectomy means removal of the lamina of a vertebra so that the spinal canal is completely decompressed; this approach was once used for disc excision but it is now reserved for more extensive operations inside the spinal canal. Disc excision is usually carried out through a more limited exposure in which the ligamentum flavum is removed with only a small portion of the adjacent lamina.

941 Spondylolisthesis means the slippage of one vertebral body forwards on the one below, usually at the L5/S1 or L4/5 levels. Spondylolysis is a break in the pars interarticularis and is one of the causes of a spondylolisthesis. Spondylosis means osteo-arthritic changes of the spine and is the most common of these three conditions.

942 Posterolateral fusion, possibly combined with root decompression, is the most common surgical procedure. Some surgeons advocate a more radical approach in which the deformity is reduced after a major soft tissue release followed by fusion in the reduced position. However, spondylolisthesis need not be treated unless the slip is progressing or it is causing pain.

943 The most common type of scoliosis is the adolescent idiopathic type. This condition usually affects girls and produces a progressive curve, convex to the right, in the thoracic region. It is a particular problem because it can develop rapidly, producing an ugly rib hump at an age when girls are particularly sensitive about their appearance.

944 The patient should be nursed flat on pillows and rolled regularly on to his side. The pelvis and thorax are moved as one so that no twisting strain is put on the damaged area. Various special beds are available which make regular turning easier.

945 In rheumatoid arthritis the neck may be unstable, leading to cord injuries during intubation and anaesthesia. In particular atlanto-axial subluxation can occur leading to cord transection by the odontoid process. Therefore careful pre-operative assessment is essential.

946 An unstable injury of the cervical spine should be reduced and then the reduction maintained. Reduction is usually obtained and held by skull traction. A

halo-jacket apparatus may later be substituted to permit mobilization. Sometimes internal fixation is used.

947 If patients recover from the shock of the original injury they soon become affected by chronic urinary infection, contractures of the affected limbs, and by pressure sores. The death of such patients was often extremely unpleasant, associated with infection from sores or from urine. If breathing was affected by the injury, then pneumonia was another major cause of death.

The shoulder and arm

948 The arm is held abducted and appears longer than the opposite side. The rounded outline of the shoulder disappears because the humeral head is displaced and instead there is a sharper angulation caused by the prominent acromion. There is a fullness of the subcoracoid region where the humeral head comes to rest. Movement is not possible at the shoulder in an acute dislocation.

949 Approximately one-third of total shoulder movement occurs at the scapulothoracic articulation and the remaining two-thirds at the glenohumeral joint. This means that even after arthrodesis of the glenohumeral joint there is still a useful range of movement at the shoulder.

950 The rotator cuff is composed of the tendons of supraspinatus, infraspinatus, subscapularis and teres minor muscles. They blend with the capsule of the shoulder joint and act primarily as stabilizers of the humerus on the glenoid to allow other muscles such as deltoid and pectoralis major to work effectively. The rotator cuff muscles can act as prime movers, particularly in the early stages of abduction, but their main function is one of providing stability.

951 The circumflex nerve arises from the posterior cord of the brachial plexus. It leaves the axilla via the quadrilateral space (between teres major, subscapularis, the long head of biceps and the surgical neck of the humerus). It gives a branch to the shoulder joint and then divides into deep and superficial branches. The deep branch runs round the neck of the humerus and penetrates deltoid to supply it. A small patch of skin over the tip of the shoulder has sensory supply from this nerve. The superficial branch supplies teres minor and then becomes superficial at the posterior border of deltoid and becomes the upper lateral cutaneous nerve of the arm.

952 If the lateral view of a shoulder is unclear it is useful to
have an axial view, in which the x-ray tube is placed in
the axilla and a plate exposed on the superior aspect.
This will show the humeral head articulating with the
glenoid and can rule out dislocation. If the shoulder is
very painful a film can still be obtained without
abduction of the arm being necessary. The patient is
simply tilted back 20 degrees and a satisfactory picture
can be obtained without causing pain.

953 To a cursory examination, the shoulder is not
obviously abnormal in posterior dislocation as the
displaced head is concealed as compared with its
prominence in anterior dislocation. In addition, this
dislocation commonly occurs following electrocution or
epilepsy so that the patient is unlikely to be in a fit
state to complain of pain in his shoulder. Furthermore,
a plain PA x-ray may not show the dislocation while a
lateral may well be unsatisfactory because of overlying
shadows of the thorax—an axial view is needed.

954 Reduction of a dislocated shoulder should be as gentle
as possible to avoid further damage to soft tissues. In a
fresh injury this should be easy, but after a few days
the soft tissues become tight and open reduction may
be required. In the acute case some patients will
spontaneously reduce if they are laid prone with the
injured arm dangling over the side of the bed. Most
require manipulation under sedation or under general
anaesthesia, and muscle relaxation. The two popular
methods of manipulation are Kocher's manoeuvre and
the Hippocratic method. In Kocher's manoeuvre the
surgeon applies traction in lateral rotation and 30
degrees of abduction. The limb is then adducted and
internally rotated simultaneously and this should
obtain reduction. In the Hippocratic method the
surgeon pulls on the arm and with his stockinged foot
guides the head of the humerus into position. This
method does not consist of yanking as hard as possible
against the counter-pressure of the surgeon's foot in
the armpit. If reduction is not achieved by closed
methods there is no shame in resorting to open
reduction which is a great deal safer than repeated
forceful closed manipulation.

955 Recurrent dislocation of the shoulder is usually
secondary to an initial traumatic dislocation. In the
original injury the anterior capsule of the shoulder was
injured and the glenoid labrum torn away from the
bone leaving a defect, the so-called Bankart lesion.
This sharp edge of glenoid can make a dent in the
humeral head which is known as a Hill-Sachs lesion.
In external rotation and abduction the shoulder is
likely to slip out of joint if these lesions are present.

Surgical repair consists of an anterior approach to the shoulder and a procedure to tighten up the capsule and repair the Bankart lesion.

956 Usually this is a trivial fracture which will heal if supported in a triangular sling and if mobilization is allowed as soon as pain permits. The other common method of treatment is a figure-of-eight bandage to hold the shoulders back and so, hopefully, to reduce deformity. This is an uncomfortable treatment and is only necessary if cosmesis is particularly important to the patient. Open reduction and internal fixation is very rarely indicated.

957 Although this fracture is generally thought of as being trivial it must be remembered that a number of vital structures can be injured. The great vessels of the root of the neck, the brachial plexus and the trachea can all be damaged. Sir Robert Peel fell off his horse and a sharp fragment of clavicle lacerated the subclavian vein. He died from loss of blood.

958 Totally different principles of treatment are involved in the two types of sling. A collar-and-cuff sling supports the arm from the wrist, applying traction to the upper arm and is therefore used for fractures of the humeral shaft. Conversely, a long arm sling supports the arm under the elbow and so would cause angulation of a humeral shaft fracture, but it is useful to rest an injured shoulder, a fractured clavicle or a subluxed acromioclavicular joint.

959 'Frozen shoulder' is an adhesive capsulitis of the shoulder joint. There is thickening and fibrosis of the joint and the capacity of the capsule is markedly reduced so that there is restriction of movement in all directions. It may be post-traumatic but in other cases the aetiology is unclear.

960 In this condition, a segment of the arc of abduction is painful, while the rest of the arc is pain free. It is caused by a degenerate or inflamed area of the supraspinatus tendon being squeezed between the humeral head and the acromion during this segment of abduction.

961 There is a variety of operations, none of which is satisfactory. Osteotomy of the glenoid or humerus may give relief of pain but is not always effective. Arthrodesis will produce a pain free joint with some movement remaining at the scapulothoracic joint but sound fusion may be difficult to achieve and the stiffness may well be unacceptable in the rheumatoid patient. Total shoulder replacement has been tried but may fail due to loosening of the prosthesis or from

dislocation. Finally, an interposition arthroplasty using fascia or a silastic cup has been proposed.

962 Colles' fracture occurs most commonly in the elderly female and is usually caused by a fall on the outstretched hand. There is a fracture of the distal radius with shortening, dorsal displacement and angulation—the dinner fork deformity. Often there is an associated fracture of the ulnar styloid.

963 The aim of treatment in Colles' fracture in the elderly is to preserve movement and function—restoration of exact alignment is a secondary aim. If there is more than 20 to 30 degrees of dorsal angulation the fracture is manipulated under local or general anaesthesia and reduction is held with a plaster back slab reaching from the upper forearm to the metacarpal necks. The manipulation consists of disimpaction by traction, exaggeration of the deformity to align the dorsal cortices, and then volar and ulnar manipulation. The plaster should hold the wrist in moderate palmar flexion and ulnar deviation with pronation of the forearm. Swelling of the fingers is prevented by elevation in a high sling for a few days and by encouraging early use of the fingers, elbow and shoulder. The plaster is completed once swelling is subsiding, and x-rays should be taken at one and two weeks after injury to check that the reduction is maintained. At about six weeks after injury the fracture will have united and mobilization out of plaster can begin.

964 A Monteggia fracture-dislocation is a fracture of the upper third of the ulna with dislocation of the radial head. Sometimes the radial head dislocation is missed as the x-ray may not quite include the whole length of the bone. It is unusual for only one bone in the forearm to be fractured so that damage to the proximal or distal joints must be carefully excluded.

965 This fracture is well known for producing the disastrous complication of Volkmann's ischaemic contracture. The brachial artery can quite easily become occluded or divided, so very careful observation is needed to detect ischaemia early. If it is detected, operation to decompress the artery and the fascial compartments must be performed immediately.

The hand

966 The deep flexor tendons act on the terminal phalanges of the digits and function is tested by active flexion of the terminal interphalangeal joint while the examiner immobilizes the rest of the finger. The superficial flexor tendons insert into the middle phalanges and are

tested by asking the patient to flex one finger at a time while the others are kept straight by the examiner, a manoeuvre which eliminates the mass action of the deep flexor.

967 The median nerve supplies the radial side of the palm of the hand, the palmar surface of the radial three and a half digits and the dorsal aspect of their terminal phalanges. The ulnar nerve supplies the ulnar one and a half digits and the ulnar side of the hand on both the dorsal and palmar aspects. The radial nerve supplies the dorsal aspect of the radial side of the hand and the proximal part of the dorsal aspect of the radial three and a half digits. There is considerable variation in the sensory innervation and also a good deal of overlap which may become apparent if one nerve is injured.

968 The skin becomes dry and warm and feels smooth to the touch. Dirt does not stick to dry skin as easily as moist skin and this may show up the denervated area on the radial side of the hand. There is wasting of the thenar eminence and loss of power of abduction of the thumb. Provided the nerve injury is a low one there will be no impairment of the long flexors but pinch grip is likely to be affected.

969 The hand lies in a characteristic posture of clawing of the little and ring fingers due to paralysis of the intrinsic muscles. The hand is markedly wasted, especially the hypothenar eminence and on the dorsal aspect between the metacarpal bones. There is loss of abduction and adduction of all the fingers but the intrinsic muscles most easily tested are the first dorsal interosseous muscle which normally abducts the index finger, and abductor digiti minimi which abducts the little finger. There is sensory loss over the ulnar side of the hand and the ulnar one and a half digits.

970 Abductor pollicis brevis is innervated by the median nerve in at least 99 per cent of subjects. It is tested by laying the hand on a flat surface with the palm up. The patient is asked to lift the thumb straight up away from the palm and this power is tested against resistance.

971 The main deficit is loss of finger and wrist extensor function. It is difficult to open the hand enough to grasp large objects, but the power of grip is also weakened. The sensory deficit on the back of the arm and hand is not usually a major problem.

972 There are four main types of grip—the power grip, in which all the fingers close round the gripped object; the chuck grip, involving the thumb, index and middle fingers and which gives fine control of movements as

when holding a pen; the pinch grip, between the pulp of the index finger and thumb; and the key grip, between the tip of the thumb and the radial side of the index finger.

973 The blood supply of the scaphoid can only enter via a strip of bone on the dorsal aspect of the waist of the bone as a large proportion of its surface is covered in articular cartilage. A fracture across the waist of the scaphoid incurs a considerable risk of avascular necrosis of the proximal fragment of bone.

974 In trigger finger there is a tendency for the finger to become stuck in full flexion. It can be extended either by active effort or by passive extension when it becomes free with a snap. The long flexor tendons catch in the fibrous flexor sheaths at the level of the distal palmar crease which may be due to tightness of the sheath, thickening of the tendon, or proliferation of local synovium, the cause of which is usually unknown.

975 Elevation of the limb is an effective way of minimizing oedema and is best achieved by using a roller towel at the side of the bed. If a sling is worn the hand must be kept high. Movement is very important in pumping away oedema fluid and so preventing stiffness, so early movement should be encouraged. Infection is a very potent cause of stiffness and drainage of any infection and treatment with antibiotics should be particularly vigorous in the hand.

976 Total loss of either power or sensation in the hand is a serious disability but loss of sensation is particularly crippling. The affected hand is liable to repeated injury and infection. Provided the arm is able to place a paralysed hand it can still perform an important function if sensation is normal.

977 This injury, which occurs most commonly in young men, causes localized pain and tenderness over the anatomical snuff box. Most fractures are undisplaced and often not detectable on the x-ray taken shortly after the injury. If strongly suspected clinically, treatment should be started even if x-rays are normal—this consists of immobilization in plaster from the forearm to the metacarpal heads including the thumb. Repeat x-rays at 10 days, including oblique views, will usually demonstrate the fracture if present. Healing takes from 8 to 12 weeks on average but non-union and avascular necrosis of the proximal pole sometimes occur, when operative treatment needs to be considered.

978 Most such fractures can be treated by splintage to the adjacent finger and encouraging early movement. Stable fractures must be differentiated from the unstable for which other forms of treatment are required.

979 Bennett's fracture is really a fracture-dislocation of the base of the thumb. A blow on the metacarpal causes a fracture through the base of the bone extending into the joint. Usually a small triangular piece of bone is left in its normal place and the rest of the bone is subluxated or dislocated laterally.

980 The area known as 'no-man's land' is between the distal palmar crease and the middle phalanx of the digit. In this area the deep and superficial flexor tendons lie within a fibrous sheath and are very likely to form adhesions. For this reason orthodox teaching was that no man should perform a primary repair of flexor tendons in this region.

981 This is in the middle of no-man's land and primary repair can easily lead to severe adhesions. Primary repair is acceptable treatment, but only if it is performed under the best possible conditions. In other words the wound should be fresh and caused by a sharp instrument with no crushing or gross contamination of tissue. In addition the surgeon should be experienced in tendon surgery and have the right equipment to perform it. If there is doubt on any of these scores it is better to go for early wound healing and mobilization of the finger, and a secondary tendon graft at a later date.

982 Infections are more damaging in the hand than elsewhere because they quickly lead to swelling and stiffness. Fibrosis around a focus of infection, while causing little functional effect in most parts of the body, may profoundly upset the function of the hand.

983 Treatment of pus in the hand should be vigorous and early—this includes both drainage of pus and full antibiotic therapy. The hand should be elevated and mobilized early to reduce oedema and to prevent stiffness.

984 The key factors are maintenance of mobility and the avoidance of infection. The best way of achieving these two aims is to clean the wound, dress it with silver sulphadiazine cream and enclose the hand in a loose polythene glove. Locally applied dressings are less satisfactory as they tend to prevent movement.

985 A grease-gun injury occurs when lubricant is accidentally injected into the hand under pressure and

requires early and vigorous treatment. The injected
material spreads in the tissue planes and may end up a
long way from the injection site producing a lot of
swelling and fibrosis. Treatment consists of early
surgical excision of all injected material. Other
industrial materials such as oil or paint may be
involved in this type of injury.

986   This injury almost always occurs from punching
someone in the mouth. The cut may be small but is
very likely to be highly contaminated and there is
often a piece of tooth embedded in the wound. It is
important to treat this injury seriously and perform a
complete surgical debridement and to give full doses of
antibiotics. The metacarpophalangeal joint is likely to
be involved and sepsis here will produce a very
awkward stiff finger.

987   Usually the patient first notices pain and tingling in
the radial three and a half digits although it often
includes the whole hand and may spread up the arm as
far as the shoulder. The symptoms tend to be worse at
night, often wakening the patient, and may be relieved
by hanging the arm over the side of the bed. If
symptoms persist, motor changes are likely to occur
with wasting of the thenar eminence and weakness of
abductor pollicis brevis. The patient often complains of
a tendency to drop things.

988   De Quervain's syndrome comprises pain over the
tendon sheaths of flexor pollicis brevis and abductor
pollicis longus with palpable thickening. It is due to
stenosing tenovaginitis of the tendon sheaths at the
radial styloid. It may be helped by local injection of
steroids but surgical release is usually required.

989   Dupuytren's disease occurs most commonly in men
aged over 40, sometimes in association with chronic
liver disease. It usually starts with thickened nodules
of fibrous tissue in the palms of the hands and this
extends into the little and ring fingers to cause
progressive contractures of the metacarpophalangeal
and proximal interphalangeal joints. Progression is
usually very gradual but in some patients, particularly
the younger ones, it can be more aggressive and cause
multiple severe contractures. There are frequently
pads of tissue on the dorsal aspect of the finger joints
and nodules of Dupuytren's tissue are sometimes found
on the soles of the feet.

990   A ganglion is a cyst arising from a synovial cavity,
either a joint or a tendon sheath, usually about the
wrist. They are smooth and fluctuant and contain
clear, glary fluid. They are often asymptomatic but if

they give trouble they can be excised although there is
a chance of recurrence.

What is . . .?

991   A cyst is a collection of fluid in a sac lined by
       epithelium or endothelium. The word originates from
       the Greek word for bladder.

992   A fistula is an abnormal track connecting two
       epithelial surfaces.

993   A sinus is a blind track leading away from an
       epithelial surface into surrounding tissues, and lined
       by granulation tissue.

994   An ulcer is a defect in an epithelial surface due to
       progressive cellular destruction rather than sudden
       trauma.

995   A carbuncle is an area of subcutaneous gangrene, due
       to staphylococcal infection. The lesion most
       commonly occurs at the back of the neck.

996   An empyema is a collection of pus in the pleural
       cavity. The term is also used for an abscess in an
       obstructed hollow viscus, particularly the gall
       bladder or appendix.

997   'Felon' is a term sometimes used for an acute
       suppurative infection in the pulp overlying the
       terminal phalanx of a finger—its importance lies in
       its tendency to lead to osteomyelitis of the
       terminal phalanx.

998   In a case of obstructive jaundice, if the gall bladder is
       palpable, then the jaundice is not due to stones in the
       common bile duct.

999   Sister Marie-Joseph's nodule is a secondary deposit
       seen in the umbilicus in cases of intra-abdominal
       malignancy.

1000 Editors' comment: Throwing an obscure name at you
       is a ploy beloved of examiners. If Gazornenplat wasn't
       the middle European inventor of a variety of
       pyloroplasty, jejunostomy or herniorrhaphy, then
       beware—having noted your Alma Mater, the
       examiner may be inviting you to hang yourself by
       showing total ignorance of the name of your recently
       retired Professor of Surgery, a phenomenon all too
       common amongst generations of medical students!

Pocket Examiner in Medicine

Alex Lawrence, MB, ChB, MRCP(UK)
Zachary Johnson, MRCPI, DTM & H, DCH, DPH, DObst

1st edition 1983

This comprehensive aid to revision for vivas in clinical medicine contains questions and answers on:

Cardiovascular system / Respiratory system / Alimentary tract, liver and pancreas / Nervous system / Kidney function and disorders; water, electrolyte and acid-base balance / Endocrine and metabolic disorders / Bone and calcium metabolism / Infectious diseases and immunization / Veneral diseases / Haematology / Immunology, autoimmune disease and rheumatology / Muscle disorders / Dermatology / Iatrogenic disease / Poisoning and overdoses / Genetics / Nutrition / Multisystem disorders

210 × 99 mm / 382 pp
Limp / 0 272 79696 4

Pocket Examiner in Regional and Clinical Anatomy

Peter Abrahams and **Matthew Thatcher**

1st edition 1981

This comprehensive aid to revision for anatomy vivas contains questions and answers on:

Head and neck / Upper limb / Thorax / Abdomen / Pelvis and perineum / Lower limb / Back

Bibliographical notes on eponyms and extensive references are given.

210 × 99 mm / 284 pp
Limp / 0 272 790621 2

Pocket Examiner in Obstetrics and Gynaecology

Peter Bowen-Simpkins, Consultant Obstetrician and Gynaecologist, Singleton Hospital, Swansea
David H O Pugh, Senior Registrar, University Hospital of Wales, Cardiff

1st edition 1983

This comprehensive aid to revision for obstetrics and gynaecology vivas provides question and answer practice for both private study and discussion. It is designed to supplement standard texts and every question is referenced to a relevant section from one of the better known obstetrics and gynaecology textbooks.

Contents: Questions – Obstetrics: Basis of Antenatal care / Assessment of fetal wellbeing / Antenatal disorders / Normal labour / Disorders of labour / Puerperium / The neonate / Epidemiology / Questions – Gynaecology: Anatomy of the female reproductive organs / Physiology of menstruation / Disorders associated with the menstrual cycle / Intersex / Amenorrhea, virilism and hirsuitism / Abortion, ectopic pregnancy and trophoblastic disease / Disease of the vulva / Diseases of the vagina / Disease of the cervix / Disease of the uterus / Disease of the fallopian tubes / Diseases of the ovaries / Endometriosis / Uterine displacements, prolapse and associated urinary problems / The climacteric and menopause / Answers – Obstetrics / Answers – Gynaecology / Index

210 × 99 mm / 256 pp
Limp / 0 272 79695 6

Pocket Examiner in Physiology

Mary L Forsling, BSc, PhD, Senior Lecturer, Department of Physiology, Middlesex Hospital Medical School, University of London

1st edition 1981

This comprehensive aid to revision for physiology vivas provides question and answer practice for both private study and discussion. It is designed to supplement standard texts on physiology and every question is referenced to a relevant section from one of the better known physiology textbooks.

Contents: Preface / Some physiological variables and their approximate values in SI units / SI conversion table / Key to references and further reading / Questions / General physiology and body fluids / Systems of the body / Co-ordinated functions of the body systems / Answers

210 × 99 mm / 180 pp
Limp / 0 272 79635 2

Pocket Examiner in Pharmacology

Tirza Bleehen, BSc, MSc, PhD, Lecturer in Pharmacology, The Middlesex Hospital Medical School, University of London

1st edition early 1983

This comprehensive aid to revision for pharmacology vivas provides questions and answers on: Principles of drug action, pharmacokinetics, pharmacodynamics / General pharmacology / Peripheral nervous system / Central nervous system / Cardiovascular / Renal drugs / Gastrointestinal drugs, drugs acting on blood, vitamins / Endocrine drugs / Chemotherapy of infections / Chemotherapy of neoplastic diseases

210 × 99 mm / 272 pp
Limp / 0 272 79645 X

Pocket Examiner in Biochemistry

D G O'Sullivan, Reader, Courtauld Institute of Biochemistry, The Middlesex Hospital Medical School, University of London

1st edition 1983

This comprehensive aid to revision for biochemistry vivas provides question and answers on:

Acids and bases / Amino acids and peptides / Investigation techniques / Proteins, structure and function / Oxygen-transporting proteins / Enzymes / Some important types of substrate molecule / Glycolysis and fatty acid oxidation / Citric acid cycle, electron transport and oxidative phosphorylation / The fed state / The fasting state / Amino acid metabolism / Nucleotide metabolism / Nucleic acids and protein synthesis / Lipids and steroids / Control of metabolism / Mineral metabolism / Liver and bile / Blood and urine / Biochemistry of tissues / Metabolism of foreign compounds

210 × 99 mm / 224 pp
Limp / 0 272 79644 1

Pocket Examiner in Endocrinology

Mary L Forsling, BSc, PhD, The Middlesex Hospital Medical School, University of London

1st edition early 1984

This comprehensive aid to revision for vivas in endocrinology contains questions and answers on:

Neuroendocrinology / Endocrine control of metabolism / Reproductive endocrinology / Salt and water balance / Endocrine function of tissues not classically part of the endocrine system

210 × 99 mm / 168 pp
Limp / 0 272 79682 4